Finding my

DELICIOUS

Leeorah Hursky

ISBN :978-0-9804705-4-3

Cover Art and design. Leeorah Hursky

Dedication

To Scott Foster

FOREWORD BY SCOTT FOSTER

Kitchen therapy is about understanding and developing a better relationship of how we nourish our bodies and explore the emotional issues that have been holding us back. Practical food skills combined with a therapeutic process help to heal fractured relationships with food and self.

Leeorah Hursky presented to me as a woman in a state of defeat. Years of grappling with her views of food and self-loathing, had all come to a point where she needed help to explore why she viewed herself and what she consumed, in such a negative way.

Leeorah had grown up in a household where food was a commodity.

A house where food was used to punish.

A house where children were not allowed to be part of the food preparation process.

A house where treats were kept under lock and key.

A house that normalised shame around consumption, appearance and social standing.

A house that never really felt like a home.

At the beginning of Leeorah's journey we explored the 'trigger foods', the 'disliked foods' and the 'foreign foods'. She worked on developing a relationship with foods that bought up negativity for her. We challenged old notions around taste, texture and feelings towards certain foods. We explored old taste memories and presented her with new and flavoursome combinations and re-looked at these old 'enemies' as potential new friends. We explored the tactile nature of food, discarding kitchen utensils in favour of getting our hands 'dirty' and allowing the exploration of the deprived inner child, to feel food again. We explored how we eat. Who we eat with. The language that happens over a dinner table, the giving and receiving of food and most importantly the mental thought process around consuming, absorbing and what nourishment it gives to a person.

Leeorah learnt to cook. Through months of challenging herself and stepping outside her very narrow comfort zone, she learnt to experience the joy and love of all aspects of food. Sourcing food, holding food, smelling food, storing food, pairing foods, touching foods, cooking foods and really tasting foods. She came so far on her journey that she rebuilt her kitchen in her home. A space that she now feels comfortable in and relishes in her new-found love. Food was no longer just fuel.

Along the pathway to discover what foods resonated the most with Leeorah, we hit some stumbling blocks. These presented in the form of foods that bought up a visceral reaction upon seeing, smelling, touching or tasting certain foods. The reaction was so strong we chose to deviate from the practical skills around food and explore the body-held traumas that were associated around these foods and triggers.

Leeorah was open and willing, no matter how

traumatic the memories, to explore what had happened to her as a child, that brought up such strong repulsive reactions.

We worked on reliving old memories that had manifested in the body over years of suppression. We explored the child that was Leeorah and looked into her world of trauma, neglect and self-protection.

After many tears and confronting scenarios were explored and an understanding of why she has lived her life as she has, a point of peace and resonance was reached.

Once Leeorah had faced her story she was able to draw on her understanding of her past, she was able to look at how she wanted her future to be. Once she had developed an understanding of what a healthy boundary was, she was able to impose them on herself and others. Once she understood how food can be the source of life both physically and mentally, she understood how she could move forward to being the best version of herself.

Leeorah was a joy to walk alongside. She was open to the process, practised the process and is now living the rewards of the process. A fierce loving soul about to embark on living her best life with food as her friend.

Chapter 1: Kitchen Therapy

I always said I needed a kitchen therapist to retrain me how to cook and eat. I actually did not know that there was such a person in this world. I have had food and cooking issues all my life. I finally met a person like this - Scott Foster is a chef as well as a counsellor - the perfect person to take me on the journey of entering the kitchen and delving into the darkest corners of my being.

He has taught me the basics of cooking. (Keep in mind I was never allowed in the kitchen as a child.) He has taught me how to play with different herbs and spices and how not to be afraid of being in the kitchen. He has also taught me to be adventurous with food, introducing foods that I would not touch (I kid you not, salads and vegetables). He has taught me that even great chefs make stuff-ups and it's ok to dump the food.

His approach in the kitchen is one of love and absolutely no judgement. The fact that I still hold a knife like a paint brush does not phase him. He is love in action in the kitchen and he imbues me with that love. He is a highly sensitive person and I have total trust in him that he knows what he is doing.

His approach was hands-on in the kitchen, allowing my phobias about food to surface. Allowing my fear of certain foods to present. It had nothing to do with the actual food but all about my childhood traumas. Some of the reasons why I go green at aubergine might never be understood, or as I discovered later on, I had perfect reason to be abhorred by this vegetable.

What I did uncover is that I was force-fed as a baby.

It has never been about food but about all the trauma that was suppressed.

When I first arrived at Scott's house, I wanted to only learn Ayurvedic cooking. He told me upfront that that was not his style and he could refer me to someone who was an Ayurvedic teacher. I soon realised that that and all other diets, Keto, vegan, vegetarianism are all in the same boat: DISORDERED EATING. Mainly under a so-called healthy name. The core is all the same: self-harm of one sort or another, anorexia, cutting, obesity, health obsessions.

I arrived at Scott's house early in 2021. I was a total wreck of a person. In his words, totally depleted. I, of course, still believed I was coping. But a lifetime of being the tough cookie had taken its toll on me.

Physically I was depleted, with weird body aches and pains and fevers to boot. I had had many medical investigations to see what was physically wrong with me. Emotionally I was dried up. Years of over-giving had taken its toll on me.

At our first session he explained how he worked. For me that was unnecessary as I knew I needed him. I had had a very unhealthy relationship with food, with cooking and especially with the kitchen.

I would walk into a kitchen and pots would fall

down. I had traumatised my children with my cooking and the final straw was when I burnt water at my daughter's house. Yes, a hard act to follow.

The kitchen was a place of pure stress for me. All kitchens fell in that category.

My relationship to food was that I just had to eat to stay alive. There was no love at all. (Bar chocolates and sugar, which were my crutches in life.) I said if I could live on chocolates and ice cream I would be happy. That certainly was not a healthy combination for a diabetic.

I had spent 60 odd years on various diets and always food came with a big NO. No cream, no oil, no butter, just a list of nos. I could add no pleasure through eating or cooking.

I continued to be heavy all my life. In my head I was always fat. Yet looking back at pictures, at times I had the perfect body. I was unhappy with my body constantly. Not surprisingly, I got diabetes with all the hate I fed my body.

I had no clue how to nourish myself at all. I was a junk-food eater and I was into junk sex and had a hedonistic (pleasure-seeking) lifestyle whenever I could manage it.

At the first session it was declared that the word diet, fat and kilos were banned and were never to be spoken about again. Such a relief that was.

One of my biggest traumas (little did I know then that more were to come) was the rejection of me by my mother. It seemed that she actually hated me.

That was the hardest pill to swallow. The heaviest burden I was carrying on my shoulders. Or so I believed.

My weight had nothing to do with food but with the rejection that I had tried to cover up my whole life. That I have hedonistically tried to soothe with my junk choices.

The rejection that I had suffered was then translated subconsciously to food. I said that I had food allergies but that was not the case - that was me fast-forwarding the rejection I had swallowed onto food. The hatred I was putting onto my body via food.

I don't know if I would have had the courage to face this rejection without the support that I was receiving from Scott. And yes, at this point I am still dependent on him. It is as though I am a child learning again. Learning what healthy boundaries are, learning how to actually cook. Learning how to eat again.

My lack of boundaries had led me to over support ex boyfriends, and friends living for free in my apartment. I could not say no. I would give my time and listening ear to friends who were hooked into drama. I would also play out dramas for some friends really well. I was frantically trying to save the starving of Africa. The truth is that I was the one starving. Starving inside from lack of love, originally from my mother and then from myself.

Overcompensating by literally trying to buy love. I had come from South Africa where I was brought up by nannies who were paid to love me. I just continued that behaviour and transferred it onto men.

Men also became my projects in life. How I could transform them into these wonderful, successful men. The energy and money that went into these attempts is actually quite sickening.

I have since let go of all those attachments including saving Africa. And it feels like an amazing release. In this journey I have had to let go of most friendships as they too were built on shaky grounds. I am happy to have a few special people who have survived my culling.

My first sessions in the kitchen were anxiety-filled. I mean, the kitchen was my enemy, not my friend. Scott was joyfully always there in total support and love and no judgement at all. In a short while I started to create exotic meals and actually enjoyed the kitchen to such a degree that I decided to renovate my existing kitchen.

This small renovation then turned into a whole house renovation, and all because I started to like cooking. Little did I know to what extent my whole body would go through with this renewal of self.

I see the renovation on a bigger scale. It is the full renovation of me. It is not only the renovation of my kitchen (heart) but of my bathroom (womb) (this had to be done twice), my lounge room (upper body) and my deck (lower body).

I know working this way and seeing things differently to most, I am able to get through this phase and soon I will be in a magnificent kitchen creating gorgeous meals again.

My daughter, who is an award-winning kitchen

designer, has designed the whole project and it is a labour of love between us. Even though she is in London, she is overseeing it all. I also have a builder who works well with me. As someone recently said, I have an ability to call in great builders. I did mess up with the tiler but hey one mistake in the whole picture is minor.

Before the renovation started, and I was into my kitchen therapy, I was happy to prepare a meal that took two hours to create and then to serve guests. That was something new for me. It was at one of the gatherings that I had, that most of the guests turned around and said I was a great cook. It was a shock to my ears as that was the furthest thing I would think of myself. And yet there it is - under all that, I am emerging as a great cook. Whoever would have thought that was possible?

And so it is I am uncovering in me a new love of cooking, of being able to cook with cream and butter and everything that was previously forbidden in my life.

And I am also happy to play with recipes and create. Recently I created a cake for my builder who was allergic to everything - it was a great achievement, especially since it was not about any of my allergic reactions.

It has been a journey welcoming back things that were forbidden for so long and allowing them into my life again. And yes, metaphorically as well. It is allowing love back into my life, especially from me to me in a wholesome way.

And finally, how do I integrate the rawest rejection I had?

Well, there is gratitude.

Gratitude that I became a strong cookie from early on.

Gratitude that I can cope on my own.

Gratitude that I have a can-do attitude.

Gratitude that I am incredibly brave on many fronts.

And finally, major gratitude to Scott who has held my hand as I regrow me.

One day I will be able to let go of his hand. Until then there will be many more kitchen adventures.

The chapters that follow are my writings before and after sessions with Scott; this helped to solidify my learning and to bring about the healing that was so essential.

Things I learnt from Scott

There were bitter pills for me to swallow on this journey. It was always the sugar/chocolates that I ran to in order to bring some comfort to me. That behaviour continued all my life, whilst not actually knowing what I was running from.

Some have asked me to write recipes. Honestly that is way beyond my scope as mainly I now play in the kitchen without recipes.

However, I will share snippets of what I learnt from Scott.

Have boundaries.
This was a big one for me as I was so open to anyone and anything, plus I had a trusting naivety.

I have learnt to say no even if it is uncomfortable.

This is a tough one to learn and to practice but I see now it gives me security that I am trustworthy, even to myself.

Chapter 2: My Childhood

Last night I watched the movie for the second time 'To the bone' on Netflix and it deeply touched me. It was the story of an anorexic young woman.

I am not anorexic yet I carry the same blueprint.

I have been overweight all my life yet the underlying issue is the same as an anorexic: I don't deserve to eat.

My eating has always been stressed and even though I was not consuming great amounts, contrary to public opinion, I continued to be overweight.

My head's siren talk constantly was, I am fat. And this negative self-talk continued even when I was thin and gorgeous. I never saw myself as beautiful, yet in hindsight and seeing pictures of my past, I can see I was a stunner. My whole life, all I could think was that I was fat. It overrode everything - my talents were undermined by this thought, my achievements were not honoured by this thought. It was all-consuming and always there.

In the movie the mother feeds her daughter with a bottle and in a way, I crave that. To be held like a child and to be fed like a baby.

Recently at a cooking workshop where I was a participant, another student and I role played being fed as a baby. He held me as a baby and spoon fed me. My reaction was to squeeze my mouth shut. I got to see that as a child I had been force-fed, with no love.

As an adult, even now I wanted to be fed like a

baby. Held lovingly in a lap and be fed. And no, Scott never did that!

It has been a life long journey to come to a place of peace with the kitchen, with food, with love for me. It is a work in progress.

I have had what appears to be a very fortunate life and for that I am grateful. However, it did come with some major monsters I have had to face.

I grew up in apartheid South Africa when apartheid was rife. I had nannies doing my mother's work and I was never allowed into a kitchen. As a child I was pretty much in the care of the nanny. I never had to pick up my clothes off the floor or make a bed, let alone cook. I was a spoilt white South African child. There, this was common whilst I was growing up.

I grew up in the seaside village of Muizenberg in Cape Town, with what seemed like a pretty relaxed upbringing. I had a best friend Steven and we would roam the streets and be inseparable. Until puberty of course, and then we seemed to drift apart. If my mother wanted me to wear a dress she would get Steven to persuade me to wear one. I was pretty much a wild tomboy, doing whatever my brother would do.

I remember even threatening to punch some kids for taunting my older brother. Evidently, I was more his protector than he was mine.

However, there was so much unsaid in South Africa. The Whites hated the Blacks, yet they were happy for them to bring up their children. The Blacks hated the Whites and had worked out their own revenge system.

I grew up with nannies paid to love me and a somewhat vacant mother and absent father.

So where is it that I am fortunate? Money was never in short supply and I had all my external needs met.

I learnt from an early age to be my own support system and to rely on no one.

I became tough through life and was not afraid to be an achiever. I have a "just do it" attitude to life. I still have that attitude.

In facing my monsters full on now, I look at other big personalities and I know that they did not have easy lives.

I have met with masters and have had training in the healing fields with the highest in the category. (I write about that part of my life in my book "*Naked Soul.*")

Yet over the last year I crumbled to the ground, often thinking - how was I given such gifts if I can't even heal myself? I stopped painting. I stopped dancing. And yes, it is the time of Covid so I am not alone in this sinking to the ground.

In the last year I broke contact with most people. I was too exhausted to continue to boost them up, the role I evidently took on in my persona.

It was not the healing work that drained me but the personal interactions with people. The line between the two became blurred. As though I was a therapist on tap for friends. In the healing work, in sessions, there were strict boundaries hence I was not depleted by them.

I am now learning boundaries in my day-to-day life.

It was in my collapsed state that I met the Kitchen Therapist, Scott.

He is both a chef and a therapist and if they coud clone people, he is one who should be first on the list.

There is a rise in eating disorders, cutting and addictions, with children as young as five starting with fussy eating. As the problem is food-based (seldom the cause) the solution should be food-based.

Emotional talk therapy is the long way around to sorting this out.

Ten years ago I wrote the book *Emotional Fat* with my cousin Amy. She was anorexic/bulimic and I was obese. In it I express how I would love to meet someone to retrain me how to cook and how to eat.

This was a very long manifestation - it was ten years before I met Scott. (I am much faster at manifesting builders...!)

It was on Facebook that I saw that someone had written about him. I knew immediately that he was the one.

When I first met him I was enthused that he should have a TV programme called *The Elephant in the Room*. With his own great personal boundaries, I learnt to back off. And so it is that I am writing about my journey with an eating disorder, to come to a place of acceptance and joy in the kitchen.

I am not fully healed yet but I share my journey of facing my deepest monsters that I had spent a lifetime avoiding. There will be times when these monsters are shared that will be very hard for the average reader to comprehend. It is true, it did happen and I have come out the other end. I will be sharing the rawest of the emotions of my own healing and hopefully it will help others heal. I do come to a place of love within that is precious.

It is my personal journey of being brave enough to face such heaviness.

I have found, and especially in the time of Covid, that when we face the darkness within, we find the jewel/light.

These writings are about my journey to reclaiming myself. To facing the many elephants in my room.

Things I learnt from Scott

Even great chefs make mistakes.

Ditch the food - if I mess up, it's not the end of the world.

Chapter 3: The Aubergine

I guess we all have likes and dislikes of food and added into that pot, the allergies that many people are living with.

I have seen through working with Scott that my so-called allergies were really just aspects of myself that had not been integrated. I call it little pockets of self-hatred. I am now able to eat all foods that I desire.

However, there are two foods that freak me out, still. I write about this extensively in the Fish chapter.

One of the foods of displeasure (to put it mildly) is aubergine.

Even writing the word brings an unpleasant feeling in my body.

Scott knew my food triggers and as we worked through them he got bolder, bringing in bigger triggers.

This particular session involved bringing in aubergine (I want to vomit even just writing about it.)

I started off in the kitchen with him with a gung-ho attitude, like I can now cook and nothing can phase me. Soon after cutting the aubergine he noticed me going green. He actually spotted it faster than I did.

Have I mentioned that he is highly sensitive and intuitive?

He asked what it reminded me of and my answer was a cadaver (a dead body). I had experienced cadavers at university whilst training as a Dental

Hygienist.

I mean that is a pretty harsh outlook for the humble vegetable.

We continued to cook even though I was getting greener and greener. It was whilst I was washing my hands that I had this thought - "kiss me." Now to note I am not attracted sexually to Scott and certainly there are very professional boundaries in place both ways. It was strange to have that thought and in my logical mind I thought maybe that's him and his wife in the kitchen. At the time I never even mentioned it to him as it was so left field for me whilst I was changing shades of colour fast.

I left that session with the cooked humble vegetable in a container. And was feeling sicker and sicker. It was whilst driving on the highway this suicidal thought came in, that maybe I should just swerve under a truck. A pretty radical response triggered by a simple vegetable.

The meal ended up in the bin very rapidly but I continued to feel sick for days.

At a later session I was able to verbalise the "kiss me" bit, but am not sure I even told him about thinking about swerving under a truck.

It was months into the process with Scott that I actually got to re-live the experiences associated with the aubergine and fish and they were extremely disturbing on all levels.

I don't know if I will ever get over fish and cooking aubergine but those two can now go onto my

'Fuck off' list. Never to be eaten.

Right in the beginning of this journey Scott also got me to make a 'Fuck it' list. This list is for foods that I have been denying myself all my life. It was great in the beginning - he would ask me what I enjoyed on the list. It took away the guilt of eating what was so-called bad food.

And so it is that I have been introduced to cooking with cream, and butter and oil. And eating chocolate when I want to. It is a journey that I am on and one day eating will be an enjoyable process for me.

There are still more elephants to meet but for now I know I can cook a great meal.

I am forever grateful that I met a kitchen therapist.

Things I learnt from Scott

Have a "fuck it" list.

All the things that were previously "forbidden". As we started the journey he would check in to see if I had enjoyed what was on the list.

Chapter 4: Work in progress

I mentioned that the kitchen was not my friend, neither was food.

They both became the object of my hatred.

It was misplaced hatred. I had no idea what this hatred's cause was, and I was hooked onto the belief that it's all about food. I believed, as most people do, that the food was making me fat. It was not true at all. I believed I was allergic to certain foods. Again, that was not true. It was all misplaced hatred.

The brilliance of Scott is that he uses food as a way into the underlying causes of this hatred, by bringing love to food.

He is passionate and totally in love with the kitchen, everything I was not.

In the first session it was challenging to even enter the kitchen. I could happily have sat in a corner and sucked my thumb, like a child.

With his gentle loving guidance and simplicity in the kitchen he welcomed me in. He was fully aware of how traumatic it was for me. Finally, I had found someone with whom I could share the level of deep distress related to food and the kitchen. The fact was, that even eating anything was a cause of deep distress.

Imagine that every meal you eat is stress-ridden. But because I had never found this support I was not even able to admit to myself how traumatic food was to me.

The only relief I experienced with food was when I ate chocolates or junk food. At that point it felt like some form of relief.

There is no doubt it is the same as any addiction.

All addictions are covering up some form of imbalance. To put it mildly. In my case, extreme imbalance.

My addiction just happened to be chocolates.

Food was made to be the bad guy.

The amount of head space and anxiety dished out to food, fat and kitchens was enormous. A constant negative dialogue, non-stop.

It was Scott's persistent love of the kitchen, his joy in the kitchen and his stance of no judgement that invited me into the space.

The fact that I could ask him questions as simple as how to boil rice or an egg, encouraged me to ask more questions.

As I have mentioned, growing up I was not allowed in a kitchen. I lacked all basic skills. I lacked all skills to nurture myself on any level bar the hedonistic path I took.

You might be wondering how I brought up my family when we left South Africa and left behind nannies and cooks?

There were some sad/funny experiences when I cooked for my husband's friend and the recipe called for a clove of garlic. I had no idea what this was and threw the whole garlic head into the blender. Needless to say, said friend never ate at our house again.

I had made some big bloops. The notable one was for my mentor friend. I literally mixed two cans of tinned food and presented it. It was worse than dog food. He swore never to eat at my house again. Not a bad thing as restaurants then became our go-to spot.

I was banned from many kitchens. I almost set alight a hotel when I tried to make a piece of chicken in Austria. The fire brigade was called in. They arrived to find me with burnt chicken on a fork, trying to open windows with all alarms going wild. Rather embarrassing to say the least. I was invited to eat at the restaurant any time I wanted, rather than try to cook again.

I managed to set up a lifestyle that supported my no cooking abilities. I worked for many years at a hotel in Germany where I was fed three times a day. That was very convenient.

I managed to feed my family with repeated recipes. However, my daughters' school lunches for their entire schooling years were peanut butter sandwiches.

I gave them lots of creative art and craft experience, more than good food.

It did reach a point when they were about 14 and 15 years old that my stress levels even to shop for food had reached a high point and they took over the cooking. My oldest daughter cooked, whilst the youngest helped with cleaning. I had no idea what all this stress was about, but there it was.

They remember times when I was adamant that I was going to have a party, as I did love entertaining. At the last minute I would flake out and they would have to take over and cater.

If I would say "let us cook a meal", it was a red flag for my daughters and they would step in quickly and take over.

In hindsight I see now why there was so much food stress in my life. The hell that had happened to me was placed onto food. The food was my blanket. The scapegoat of all that had happened to me.

I think one of the most touching cooking moments with Scott was when he made me a black sesame cake for my birthday.

It felt like no one had ever lovingly made me a birthday cake.

I kept making that recipe for months afterwards until I could not eat it any more.

His approach with my distorted eating, again mildly put, was to allow all foods to be eaten. This was big for someone who had said no to so many foods. No to oil, to butter, or fat. No wonder my cooking tasted like shit. Now with all these added things my cooking tastes great.

I easily swapped over to coconut sugar and maple syrup. Not once in all the time with him have I felt like I was restricting anything. On the contrary, it is the opposite. And yes, my body has changed. I have reduced dress sizes but that is not the focus so I can't even say how much weight has shifted.

I had always liked baking - it was making real food that had failed me. I now started to experiment with baking healthy cakes and biscuits. That transition was really easy for me. In the beginning I bought litres of maple syrup! However, I soon let go of that need as well.

He introduced me to eating grapefruit.

I hated grapefruit as I had done, amongst other diets, the grapefruit diet when I was young.

At first, I could only eat grapefruit with maple syrup but soon I managed without having to adding it. The day I actually craved a grapefruit was a real breakthrough.

He also taught me how to make great green beans and asparagus. I do still have to encourage myself to eat more vegetables.

It has not been a quick turnaround to now eating healthily.

I still have cravings for sweets and I can see in retrospect it is as stuff is bubbling to the surface that sweets will be my port of call.

Scott taught me how to match herbs and spices, which ones actually worked together and most importantly, how to play in the kitchen. How to not stress about a mess in the kitchen (that used to freak me out, amongst other things).

In sessions I do not take notes - I try to remember and he encourages that as it does not limit me when I am cooking at home.

There are still times when I go to sessions that I

feel nervous but I am able to tell him. I understand now why the nervous feelings would have popped up as there was so much boiling under the surface.

With my trigger foods we have reached the understanding that there is no need to bring them to the table. These foods can remain on the "Fuck off" list. They served their purpose in bringing up the terror associated with them.

Working with him has allowed me now to be honest with myself as to how deep my wounding was. I had no idea at the extent of the wounding. At no point ever in our sessions would he sugar-coat anything. If I needed to be told a truth he was forthcoming. His truth would shake me up, to look deeper at what I was avoiding.

I also had to learn boundaries and he certainly taught them to me by actually practicing them on me.

My boundary system had been knocked right out of me from an early age. I was like a puppy dog, boundless and with no control.

I have learnt and I am still learning. I check in with myself now and instead of overriding a discomfort I will honour myself and if need be, cancel appointments.

I am a work in progress.

Things I learnt from Scott

Play with combinations of foods, spices and herbs.

Experiment with condiments and herbs. I have also learnt with bigger dishes like soups to flavour small amounts. (Saves you throwing out the whole pot should you mess up!)

Chapter 5: Naja

You can't make this stuff up even though it seems so unbelievable. It is all true.

I am beyond blown away.

A few years ago, I felt like I was going to have a stroke. Seriously, all the signs were there, and by grace I came across a medical doctor/homeopath, Murray Rushmere, who understood me. It was interesting that I did not have a stroke, however my first cousin did. Was I tuning in to him? Who knows?

Murray understood me because first of all I speak a different language. Although I speak English I work on the principles of energy and speak in energy. Hard to communicate that even when writing in English. English is my first language yet the unspoken energetic energy is what I often work with, especially in the healing fields. I often look at people who don't understand me even though I am speaking English. And even worse, if I SMS people I leave out words and expect the recipient to understand me. Those close to me such as my daughter and my friend Rose fully understand me despite SMS's that look as though I am retarded. I am actually really bright if I say so myself except I am communicating with a different language and there are not many who get this language of mine.

It does become a lonely path to follow. A path I don't even try to explain to others. I do have friends trying to narrow me down on this path to write correctly and watch what I say. And so I seclude and recluse myself.

Murray understood that I could communicate energetically who I am. And he prescribed a remedy for me, which in three doses, healed me.

Fast forward two years later and I am in Australia in a place that is paradise, Byron Bay, but it is also a place that forces me inward. This town is a place of healing and to come here is to heal, not to live on a permanent basis.

It is viewed by the First Nations people as a birthing place. I have birthed a few books here.

I have been fortunate - in previous times I could work around the world and then retreat here.

Covid forced me to be stationary. I could no longer live that lifestyle of flying around the world like a gypsy. I was grounded, with the rest of the world.

And in this grounding I have once again had to look at further shadows and this time the deepest shadow of all was presented. The deepest one, or so I believed. I couldn't believe there could be deeper ones (little was I to know…)

I had a situation in my life where the tenant from hell played out, reflecting my own unfinished business. Especially reflecting the rejection my mother showed towards me.

It was the greatest change-maker of all; the outcome was that I renovated a whole house and have a new beginning.

Initially it was a really hard pill to swallow.

As I was facing this rejection I manifested body aches that were extremely intense. At one point I thought I had lung cancer, it was that excruciating. My whole body ached and it was painful to even roll over in bed. I could not bend down, nor do up my bra -everything hurt.

By the way, I have lived a very fortunate life and at 66 I did not even have a painkiller in the house.

I had to quickly make friends with painkillers and Deep Heat and various medicines.

For seven months I had been involved with my aches and pains, and had left behind my life of pleasures. I am a wild one - even at this ripe old age I could party at nightclubs and entertain young men in the true sense.

I was now hobbling like an old lady. No dancing, no partying, no painting, no writing, no sex. It was just the painkillers and me.

Just self-absorbed with the body pains.

Actually, I could not even recognise myself.

And finally, I remembered this magic homeopath, Murray Rushmere.

I have just finished speaking to Murray. First of all, it is such a relief to be understood without having to explain myself. After all he is South African and understands the upbringing of the Black nannies caring for the Whites. Even whilst the Whites are bad-mouthing all Black people. Growing up in an apartheid, racist country is hard to comprehend.

I shared with Murray my symptoms and what actually relaxed me.

A week ago I had to confront a snake above my toilet. I freaked out and had to get the builder on site to calm me down. I am afraid of snakes big time. Because of the snake and the freak out and the renovations I decided to go out of town for a few days to Brisbane.

Whilst in Brisbane, I went to a fair where there was a demonstration of snakes, and the opportunity to have one draped on you. I confronted my fear and allowed a very large python to be draped over my shoulders. Strangely enough in those moments I could actually feel my shoulders start to relax, most probably for the first time in months. The snake actually went to sleep on me and in the photos that were taken I look calm and relaxed. (Not how I was feeling inside...!)

I posted the pictures on Facebook and a friend said "Transformer... Naga goddess ... Naga Kanye..." This is what she called me. I had no idea what she meant.

These are Google's descriptions:

Naga, (Sanskrit: "serpent") in Hinduism, Buddhism, and Jainism, a member of a class of mythical semi divine beings, half human and half cobra.

Naga Kanya, also known as **"Immortal Goddess of India", "Mother Guardian" or "Snake Daughter"** is a powerful ancient Indian folklore symbol. It is believed that this snake goddess resides in the underworld with immense spiritual knowledge and power.

I shared this story with Murray and he told me

that the remedy he had given me two years previously was the snake remedy NAJA. At the time he never told me that as I would have freaked out.

You can't make this stuff up.

Amazing that my biggest fear is where my remedy is. And that I too like a snake am misunderstood, feared and avoided. And so it is that I now come into being and am becoming the NAJA/NAGA.

I am happy to report that all aches, pains and illnesses have left my body.

Things I learnt from Scott

No judgements.

Chapter 6: Shamans

I had lived a very traditional western life. I had been a dental hygienist working at universities and in private practice.

At that point of my life what you saw was what you got. I certainly did not believe in meditation or anything supernatural or spiritual.

I had enjoyed studying at university and was all for believing that what was presented was truth.

However, some things did start to surface when I was a dental hygienist - I could intuit when a patient had a disease. I was always correct as the dentist was informed and the patient had tests to confirm it.

This was rather astonishing to me - as I say, I was by the book and here was an ability that had not been taught to me. It did start to awaken in me that possibly there is more than the eye can see.

To further add to these experiences, before we emigrated to Australia, I received a body work session. I fully entered into a spiritual state and actually felt like I had levitated off the table.

Once we arrived in Australia I felt like I had come home. I had such a euphoric feeling. Finally, it felt like I could stop pretending to be the good Jewish woman. It felt like a liberation. I had never cracked the Kugel, Jewish princess scene.

I had to re-sit my dental hygiene exam in Australia and am happy to admit that I failed it as I would still be cleaning dirty teeth. That was a relief and a blessing. However, I am very grateful to my initial medical /dental training as it served me well.

At that point I decided to study naturopathy as I was now starting to move in a different direction. I enjoyed the studying and had full intentions of finishing the course.

In my first year of training I met my first Hawaiian Kahuna. I have since met four Kahunas that I know of in this life. This is a very rare privilege for a westerner. Without a doubt I have lived in Hawaii in previous lives.

The respectful name for a Hawaiian healer is Kahuna. A teacher who is a master of his trade. A sacred person honoured by his community. A title reserved for those born in the Hawaiian lineage.

They gave a demonstration of Hawaiian massage at the college I was attending. Immediately all my lights went on. There was a deep knowing of this work and an incredible desire to follow this path.

It took another six months until I could begin my training with them and my whole life turned around completely, including me leaving my husband.

I was no longer a good complying wife who believed in what you could see was real. Now a whole new world had opened up for me. I was trained to become a shaman - someone who could read more than just the body. Someone who could tap into past lives, ancestors, addictions, patterns and curses, to name a few things.

I write more extensively about this training in

other books but suffice to say that many new paths opened up for me, including the fact that I was invited to work around the world.

I was also given a healing system over three years called Akalani, which means chords or symbols to heaven.

And even with all of these great gifts and abilities, I fell flat on my face. Ill, disgruntled, in pain and unable to cook for myself.

In my journey with Scott I was very aware that he was the therapist and it was essential that he ran the show. I fully surrendered to him being the therapist.

It has been a great journey of trust. I understood really early on that he too has an ability to see more than what is presented in my words or actions. He can be present with me through hell.

He senses the slightest innuendo in my body. And although he says he is not a body worker he read my body the whole way through. He read how I would arrive with hunched shoulders or hobbling into session. Granted those qualities are obvious to see, but it was the smaller things he would read as well. Like notice me turning green long before I even knew it.

And hell I did enter and in it all I knew he was there and would help me to get through it.

The hell I had to face is more than most people could have coped with. This time entering the hell I knew I had someone holding space for me to enter it.

And I knew I trusted him to help get me out of it. It was surprising, once faced with the hell, how in a few weeks I was able to transform it.

And this whole journey with Scott began in the kitchen.

Things I learnt from Scott

Pick your battles.

Chapter 7: In this time of Covid

I operate out of the box and I do not watch news or follow mainstream information. This is a choice I make, as to be honest, I find that what comes out of the mouths of politicians and many journalists, is bullshit.

However, somehow I do know what is going on. It is on the other level where I tune in to know what is happening.

It was just before the pandemic started that I had the feeling that I needed to go back to Germany to work again. I had had a long sabbatical from healing work.

I booked a ticket and for the first time in my life as an avid traveler, I made a mistake on the departure date. I believed I was leaving at the end of February 2020. However, I had booked the ticket for the end of March.

By the time March came Covid was well and truly in and I would have been stuck in Europe for the last 2 years had I flown out in February. It was grace in action to have booked the wrong date.

I received all my money back and had to face what Covid was telling me.

So this is my personal take on it.

I sense Covid as a time of grounding. A deep call to go in and face the personal shadow. Physically at the time I was exhausted and the last thing I needed was to fly around the world. Having been grounded it was a time to go inward. Little did I know I would be doing such deep shadow work.

Energetically I see Covid as a blanket over the world. It can be used as a time of composting the dark shadow or as a time of unadulterated fear. Most of the world has gone to the fear factor, to the fear of death. As I do not fear death, working as I do in the other realms, that has not concerned me.

And in this fear of death people have grabbed onto branches and twigs to avoid death. Branches and twigs the government (or others) are dishing out in the form of toxic vaccines. With a hypnotic chant of how you are saving others. Now forgive my ignorance but when have people been concerned about their neighbours and the government concerned about the weak and elderly?

It is trying to subdue this fear with more toxins.

I am amazed at how many intelligent people have fallen for these branches instead of facing the fear of death.

And yes, I have energetically seen that the virus was started in a lab.

I do get it that people are sick and have died from it. Yet I will not buy into the toxic branch that is being offered.

I would not trust a politician to tell me how to care for my body. After all doctors have studied for years for this knowledge. They too are being bullied into submission and their innate wisdom overridden.

And yes the question is, who is feeding all this fear? Is this another import from China, to be another one of its states? After all, we import so much from China. Or are darker forces at play here? However, I take it positively and keep the premise that it is a time to face the personal dark shadow in order to emerge into the light.

Not for one moment do I trust anyone on it. This a time of division and I do not see any difference to the time of the Nazis, yet I am totally amazed how many sheep are voluntarily going to slaughter. As a Jew I can see now how it happened. How the fear and division offered led millions to their death.

I am flabbergasted how the hypnosis has affected more people than I could imagine, intelligent friends who are so called spiritual beings have taken the twig of the offering.

There is no way a trial vaccine by the world's leading crooks can be helpful to anyone.

And yet Covid time has served me so well, hearing the call on another level.

To go deep within and be composted like a flower. To go deep into my shadow. With my lifestyle previously of flitting around the world and living a life of pure hedonism, where was the time to actually face my personal demons?

It is the grace of falling so deep down that the gift of the shadow was revealed. That through the darkness I could emerge into so much light.

It took Covid, ill health, a broken spirit and guts

to emerge.

I hope that this house of cards kindly given to us will have served its purpose and will allow the new amazing light to light all beings.

Things I learnt from Scott

Have a good set of chopping knives.

Chapter 8: The next elephant in the room

I realised only recently that the stress I feel when eating, especially if around people, is that I don't deserve to eat. That belief came from the silent stares of my mother when I ate. She, after all, was svelte and beautiful and here I was, a fat, red-haired child.

I feel when I eat that I need to get the food in fast and then there is almost a relief that that duty is over. And then clean up fast as well. A stress all round.

There is no enjoyment in eating; even though I am cooking really well, there is still this stress. Also, recently I went back to cooking what I thought I had to eat. So the enjoyment went out the door even more.

Yesterday I had made a horrible cauliflower, kale and spinach dish. Most probably my three worst foods, so I tried to smother them in a cheese sauce. I did eat some but then gave myself permission to throw it out.

The duty to eat what I think I should still exists as the old diet concepts still lingers on.

My confidence in the kitchen is growing and I do know I can make a good meal. I am even enjoying cooking. Even making a mess in the kitchen and not stressing about cleaning it.

This last elephant, well I guess there could be more, is to clear the old belief that I don't deserve to eat.

In one way I think that I should have healed all this by now but I guess that it's the onion being de-layered. Also, with the great breakthrough with my mother story, I thought the food stuff would all be over.

Only chocolates or sweets would give me relief. The feeling still when I have a chocolate is that there is a relief in my body, a sweetness is back, all will be well.

I am also facing my personal relationships with people who have been important in my life.

I am in touch now with my deep sadness to lose Trent.

I met him about 30 years ago when I moved to Byron. We met on the dance floor where he gave me a spectacular wild meeting in dance. I don't think he ever danced like that with me again. We became good friends, but in fact I did not even realise he was gay. He only told me way down the track. Our friendship was wild and wacky. We laughed a lot and he sparked my creativity. He called me his muse. We hosted games nights for singles and we created a board game.

It's that connection that I talk about - to meet in creativity. I used to love it when he came around. Mainly he would come around to my house.

We had a week together on Lord Howe Island. I also had a deep spiritual event in his presence. We had been holed up in a room together because it had rained so much and I had all this pent-up sexual energy. We walked to the top of the mountain and it was there that I lay down and became one with the mountain and moved into spiritual bliss. It is hard to describe how I became one with the mountain. I was so content at that point I could have jumped off the cliff and ended my life as it felt so complete.

We were in a way like two giggling girls.

He was the one who took me to a Swinger's club and encouraged me to be serviced. That is a great friend I reckon. I have not thought about him for a while but when I do, I miss him big time.

And I believe that he misses me too. By the way he is German. However, it's his wife who is totally German in her ways.

I would like to meet him and have giggles again but it has changed so much and things were so stilted when I did see him.

Guess as I am not going to see him again, I would like to acknowledge to him how amazing it was to have a best girl/boyfriend.

Trent - we met on the dance floor where we were both sparked big time. At the time I thought you were such a good dancer, you would have no interest in me. I don't know how we moved onto being friends. We would speak on the phone often and hang out together. We would go to Mike's property and swim in the lake. Those were wonderful days. Very rich. I was not complexed about friendships at that time and had many people around me. I know people loved to hang around us. They especially loved our games nights. We laughed so much. It was a free time then. I never thought of you as boyfriend material. And then I only found out later you were gay which I guess put our friendship in a safe category.

You were there whenever I returned from my overseas trips, catching me as I came to ground in Australia.

Trent, you were a great part of my life and up to now, I have not even acknowledged it. I tried to hang onto you even after you were married but it became way too hard. Pretending to like your wife, who I don't. The harsh German who keeps you on a lead. It was too hard for me. There was no space for me. I also knew you wanted a child and to have a normal life and a hard-working woman. I never wanted a physical relationship with you - I just wanted that wild creative spark we had with each other.

I do miss you and miss that which we had.

I have had a challenging time this last year facing the rejection of my mother and in a way, it would have been good to have a friend to bounce it off with.

I know it's my rebirthing time and I guess I have to do it alone.

I miss you Trent but with these words I have to let any strands of you go from my life.

After my 67th birthday I did call Trent and asked to meet him without his wife.

It was like 25 years had not passed.

Scott, I am deeply touched by being with Trent. It is as if I want to climb into him and never let him go. As my grandchildren do with me.

I want to hold his hand all the time and physically not be parted from him. I want to snuggle up to him and feel him all the time.

And the amazing thing is that in all the time we were best friends, I never slept with him.

I think I coped with it back then, that I saw him as being gay. My coping mechanism of not being rejected.

Do you know I can't even remember - did we share a bed together? I know we did share a room together. We might have as he was the first one to point out my sleep apnea.

He is now very comfortable to call himself bisexual. I do see a big difference in him now. It is like he has stepped into his sexuality and is at ease with it. He has a new strength in him.

On our date, and we can call this our first date, I did let go fully. He ordered for me, I allowed him to drive me around. We did not have a minute of awkwardness between us.

I described us before as two giggling girls. Now I do let go of that and see him as a man standing strong.

Back then people thought we were a couple and last night we went to a ceremony together and we were taken as a couple. They saw it. Someone said we were the most loving couple she had seen. And I feel it. Others there also kept calling us a couple.

I do fully appreciate that we have never slept together as I would have thrown my traumas onto him.

His wife is doing that to him. Sounds like constantly, however she will not look at her own traumas.

I also see when he lost me he lost his sense of humour. I see the battle scars in him from his continuous battle. His mouth is now down-turned. It was not back then.

He remembers far more than me of our time together. Funnily enough he said that when we were together he never had lovers. He called us together, I guess I never saw it as that.

I like very much what I see in him now. A new strength, a new knowing who he is. He did also say that if he were free that we should still not sleep together as that would change the dynamic of what we have.

Now I wonder - is that him/or me not giving himself /myself all that we deserve in this life?

I know from previously I would want to be with him all the time. I would crave him when he was not with me.

He tells me I told him when he married her that my statement to him was that he loves a challenge. And he has had one. 25 years of constant attack.

I guess the kindest thing I did for myself was to withdraw when he married. It was kind yet hard to lose him. And it has been amazing that I could tell you that I do deeply miss him.

He is back. And who knows when I will see him again. I will not, and he knows, meet him with his wife. This is the boundary that I clearly call.

They have been to marriage therapy three times

and I do believe that this is his last attempt. He could meet me now as she was on a workshop. He is hoping this is what will get her to break through.

I of course will not interfere. But I know deeply that we both want to be in each other's lives.

We light each other up and we laugh so much. There are no secrets. He is German and I am Jewish -a tough combo but we rise above it.

For me what seems relevant now is that I have faced my deepest traumas without having to have a man poke them to the surface and I am now willing to open to love.

As it is not to be with Trent, this experience has show me that I do know how to have a fun, loving relathionship.

I open to having a fun, light, caring love relationship. One where I do not need to fight. All previous ones involved me fighting. I can clearly say it now I was fighting my own demons, and the men were coping with those unseen traumas.

I hope that the man I move forward with has Trent's qualities.

Things I learnt from Scott

Life and the kitchen are my new playgrounds to enjoy.

Chapter 9: The body does not lie

The intelligence of the body is amazing. All the time I was berating my physical body for being fat, it was being highly intelligent and protecting me. It was protecting me from the poisons that were being directed at me.

Poisons that were coming towards me energetically and physically.

It was as though the fat was an absorber of the poisons, cushioning me and protecting me. The body does wish to stay alive and this was its way of doing it.

After all, how does a child survive such abuse and stay alive?

Not only that, the body then cleverly hid these memories from me to at least keep me safe. I did have an insight once where the body was physically storing the poison in the fat cells because they could handle poison more than the other cells.

I dismissed that so quickly and went back to hating the fat body instead of praising it for its innate wisdom.

Early on in my career as a dental hygienist, when I was still in the narrow existence of what you see is what you get, I started to get information from just looking at a person's mouth. I was able to diagnose diseases in an instant. It was surprising to me and I was always correct.

It was the first clue that I had an ability that was out of the ordinary.

I also see that my training as a dental hygienist was important for the next step in my life. I was trained in the medical fields and understood the body from the western medical perspective.

I was also trained to do public speaking during my time working at dental university. I loved having 600 dentists in the palm of my hand listening to what I was sharing. My topic became how to handle the difficult child in the dental chair.

It all seems so long ago and so distant. It was merely a stepping stone.

I progressed (and share that in previous books) to working with the shamans of Hawaii where my true training took place: how to remove the root cause of illness from the body. Of course, until illness hit me and all my training went out the window and I rushed to doctors.

Now having gone through what I hope is the last of the tragic memories I welcome back my vitality.

Whilst working as a body worker I learnt early on to trust the information the body would give and never to doubt that information.

I would do a verbal interview first but usually I was looking for what they did not know, as they knew their own story verbatim and it had not helped them.

By the way, I was working internationally and never would I allow bookings prior to my arrival as I still operated as a free gypsy spirit. Those who worked with me learnt to trust that and that is saying a lot as I was working in Germany where organisation is key.

I had learnt that there are three levels we operate on: the subconscious which actually runs the show and normally we have no idea of its program, the conscious level of what we are well aware of, and the super conscious which is the higher aspect of self, the god self.

Most of the time we are operating from the lower two aspects, with the subconscious as the conductor.

In working with the clients' bodies, I was able to tap into the subconscious and it was there that change could start to happen.

Mainly I would intuit it. I do remember early on I was given visuals and during one session I saw such horrific things that both the client and I ended up screaming. It was at that point I asked not to be given visuals and so moved onto working in the feeling, intuiting range.

I implicitly trust what was given to me in a session as weird as it might have appeared. I could usually shift someone in the space of two hours without needing to see them again.

I have let go of the body work now and am in a place of "let's see what is next".

Things I learnt from Scott

Cooking is creative and fun.

Chapter 10: The chaos loop

12 October 2021

I need to write this as an honouring and a farewell to the chaos loop that has been playing out my whole life.

When I was under three, (I keep forgettig the age, even still today) my family was involved in a motor car accident. My mother was driving, and I am not sure if a tyre blew out or she hit something, but the car spun around 13 times. The nanny was flung under the car and was killed. My mother broke her spine. I was flung onto a thorn bush. Nothing happened to my father or brother. My father knew my mother had broken her spine; he stood next to her shouting that no one was to touch her. He knew that to move her would cripple her. Those words 'don't touch her' have also echoed in my life.

As I was so young and had energetically not separated from my mother, I carried the guilt and traumas and the belief that I had caused the accident. I could say I had been in an accident very factually but I had no idea of the implications it had rained on my life.

It was interesting that about 30 years later, on the exact date of the accident, the memories and the impact it had had on my life started to filter through.

One believes that a child is too young to remember. Trust me - the body holds all the information and only when the circumstances are in alignment will it release the memory.

This was shown to me again as I faced the recall of a sixty-year-old memory block. This amnesia had kept me sane from the memory of hell.

Each year at this time, I would spin into a depression or a freak out. It is amazing that the body holds the information, so accurately bringing to the surface on the exact date, the traumas that have not been resolved.

I worked with Scott on 12 October (one day before the anniversary of the accident) after I had had dreams about both my parents - a somewhat encouraging dream in which they were purchasing the hotel I worked at in Germany. The dream was an honouring of me and my work.

At our session I spoke about the accident and as Scott was talking to me I started to block everything he was saying. He is highly intuitive so I knew he knew that this was happening. He gave me the choice to work further with it or shelve it for now. I took the first option and his question to me was, why was I blocking it so intensely?

I digress here but I have to mention that I had always felt I was too much. I did one day uncover that what had happened to me was too much, not that I was too much.

Scott gave me a few minutes to reflect on why I was blocking it so intensely.

In sessions I am able to time travel back to

events.

It was the chaos of the motor accident that I did not want to enter. With his help I recalled it. The main thing in all my therapy time with him was that I felt guilty for the accident and the death of my nanny. Logically I know a two-year-old can't cause the accident, neither all this chaos, but I was feeling it. I have felt it all my life evidently.

In recent months I had also faced the fact that my mother had rejected me - a truth I spent my life running away from, with hedonistic behaviour on whatever level. Facing that was most probably the heaviest thing I have done. The thought was - if my own mother can't love me then who the hell can? It was a deeply depressing time to go through. In fact, at that point I was planning my own suicide, to end it all.

Very fortunately I was in therapy and I knew that Scott was there should it get out of hand.

Back to the session. At first I was trapped in the chaos of the accident and in the car and falling and ambulances and noises all around and feeling so guilty I had caused it. I managed to get the little girl out of the scene to take a step outside of the chaos and it was there that I saw that my mother had been in love with another man and that my birth had wrecked it all for her. Hence my feelings of guilt that I had carried to that day.

I also got to see that there was hatred towards me from her, resentment and the list goes on. The one who unconditionally loved me was the nanny who had died in the accident.

I had been carrying all that negativity as though a tube was feeding me still even though she had been dead for years. The loop was well embedded.

I was able to separate myself from my mother, and to reconnect with the love from the nanny. Freed from my mother and myself to be neutral, free for her to be able to move on to God without all the baggage and in so doing free myself to be connected to love in the true sense.

It feels like it is a rebirth of me.

To be the radiant being I was born to be.

And what do I see on the bigger picture is that WE ARE ALL TRAPPED IN A LOOP.

Mine was chaos. I look at others - I see others trapped in the self-pity loop, the ugly duckling loop, the can't have anything loop, the strangling of self loop, the arrogant loop, the princess loop, the unworthy loop and the list goes on. I believe that once one gets to the core of the loop, that is when freedom can happen.

We are in the time of Covid now, the time to face the ugly side or shady side of the self. That from which most will run, really fast. Myself included, into the world of hedonism. But I see the greatest gift in diving deep into the rejection and then seeing my personal loop and now feeling so loved and supported - granted its mainly from the unseen world at this point but that for me is real food and life. I am sure it will translate into the human world as well.

For the first time in two years I want to go and

dance tonight at a class.

Big honour and thanks to Scott for holding space whilst I moved through all that.

Things I learnt from Scott

Everything can be the canvas of life.

Chapter 11: The Fish

3 November 2021

Through all these sessions I have also been preparing myself to meet a true life partner and it was only today that I could finally verbalise all the qualities that I would like in him.

That he could match me on all levels and accept my unusualness. That he could accept the fact that I do not even know which party the prime minister belongs to and I choose to remain ignorant of what is presented in the news. That I operate on an "outside of the box" approach. That he will never suppress me. That his presence will add calm to my life yet match me creatively.

In a way that his qualities will be like my friend Shine or Trent, calm and graceful and aware and heart-centred. That love will underwrite it all. And especially that I am MET fully as I was with Papaji. (Papaji was an Indian master whom I was blessed to meet.)

However, having said all that, I still felt a tight body sensation in even thinking about meeting a partner. I am fortunate I can work through the body in reading the sensations and then facing what is under the sensations.

The emotion that was stuck was fear and it seemed around sex.

Previously I believed that my sexual appetite was my big opener; however, it was a default button that got a need met, but little else. In asking for a true meeting I finally faced the fact that it was not what I believed, sex, but something else finally that was being asked to be met. I was brave enough to face yet another elephant in the room.

Honestly, after facing the big one last time with my mother and the accident, I thought I was done and dusted.

I guess that when I am in my grave, then it will be done and dusted.

In my session today I was able to face my abhorrence of fish as well. I am not sure how these two issues presented at the same time. This abhorrence makes me feel shaky and sick.

In this session I allowed myself, through the twisting and turning in my body, to go back to a scene where I had been sexually abused.

I believe I was around the age of three or four. In this scene I could now smell and re-experience events, and yet feel totally safe in Scott's presence, knowing he could get me through it. It was also essential for me not to default to my healer role, the reason being I could easily then take over the session and for now I was the client. I finally am really learning boundaries.

In the scene I saw I was in a tin shack. The man who was abusing me, had a similar body size and features as mine. From previous visitations of this scene he inserted his grubby hands in me whilst cursing all Whites. He held me upside down like a piece of meat.

In today's scene I saw the nanny's hands were tied whilst she was watching what was happening. There was another woman watching and one cooking.

It was fish she was cooking. I re-lived the smells. I also believe there was aubergine as I have had such a strong reaction to that as well. The feeling of wanting to throw up was so strong.

After he had abused me he flung me on the floor, leaving me naked and trembling in a corner, while the group got more and more drunk. They started throwing fish at me.

I was stuck in the corner. Trembling. It went on for hours.

My body in the session was convoluting and shaking.

Scott moved the session on to what happened after the event.

I was taken by the nanny to her bathroom where I was washed. The water had blood in it. She would not look at me but carried on cursing me. Saying I was disgusting, revolting, dirty.

I was put to bed and it seems like I was in bed for a long time.

The question was where the fuck were my parents? How could they not see I had been damaged?

I was almost comatose under the sheets, my body in deep shock.

The nanny was employed for many more years.

From the age of three until eight I was sworn at and cursed daily. With a vacant mother and an absent father who would have been my role model. No wonder I was a foul-mouthed lover.

That I have survived at all is a miracle.

Scott moved the session on to me now as an adult facing the nanny.

I felt like a trapped grasshopper that had been speared. I was aware of her evil eyes piercing me. At first I could do nothing, then with his encouragement of calling an animal to help me I was able to call in the snakes. They wrapped around her. Yet her eyes were still sending daggers to me and I was still like a speared grasshopper.

He suggested I close her eyes. The snakes then covered her eyes and I started to regain some strength to kick her. Eventually I could swear at her and get the energy moving. I called in all those who love me to be around me and from that place I was able to return the disgust, the shame, the revulsion, the hate, and the guilt (as a child I believed I had done something wrong to deserve this).

There was a pool that I placed her and all who had put this stuff on me in, into that pool of revulsion. There were also a lot of dead fish. With those who loved me around me I was able to blast the shack apart.

With those who loved me around me I was able to verbalise that I would not carry all this revulsion that was bestowed on me as an innocent child. It had been my placard above my head: place your shit on me. It was all sent to a pool of revulsion which was then cleared and filled with rose water.

It has gone now. It is cleared. It is love that is now my sign above my head.

I feel so grateful to have Scott there helping as well as my ability finally to see all this revulsion I have carried for so many years. That my cells were spinning in this negative soup. And now releasing it finally to be transferred into love.

Yes, I am ready to meet my full match. This is the first time I can say it with clarity. And to him, sorry it has taken me so long to come to a new state of being.

And yes, even more surprising to me still is that I have become or am becoming a great cook. So hard to believe after a lifetime of not wanting to enter a kitchen.

Deep grateful thanks to Scott and to me for being so brave to face all these elephants finally. Liberating myself.

Things I learnt from Scott

Food was not the source of my problems. It was a result of past traumas.

Chapter 12: Celebration on two legs

16 November 2021

After each session with Scott I think - what more is there to deal with? After all I have dealt with fish being flung at me, motor accidents and rapes. The list is quite big enough, one would think, yet surprise surprise, there was more.

The session today began with me discussing my father and how he ruled the roost. Somehow, I felt that I was afraid of him. His word was it. He was a charismatic man who also happened to be extremely good looking, and had ladies always admire him. I would say that in all his adult life, he only had three months without a woman.

After my mother died of cancer, the next lady girlfriend, who he had met three months later, also got cancer. He spent seven years nursing sick women. His second wife did outlive him and she became his carer when he himself developed cancer.

I did heal my relationship with him after he had had a stroke and he told me he could hear things and see things. Finally, we were talking the same language.

My real language is energy. And even now I still surprise myself when writing, as I do not see myself as a writer. I am aware that although this is my journey it will also be other people's journeys. Those closest to me understand me even when words are not spoken.

My father also happened to be my dentist so my connection to him also was pain-filled. And trust me, I had many fillings.

I became a dental hygienist following in his footsteps. I loved being around dentists and the surgery and the buzz. I realised also I was seeking daddy connection by having teeth issues.

Later in life I became aware of how he spoke to woman, especially his second wife. It was very derogatory.

My mother was a drinker and he kept the keys to the alcohol cabinet. At 6 pm every night he would give her two drinks. The other keys were to the cupboard where the chocolates were kept. I would sneak down the stairs at midnight when all were asleep to get chocolates. Chocolates and sweets were forbidden in my house.

I swore never to do that to my daughters; at times when I could, I would have lolly jars, but because of my addiction to sugar could not maintain that.

Another set of keys were the keys to the fridge to prevent the Black servants from stealing food. What a sick environment! That's a lot of locks in one house. Everything controlled and under lock and key.

As we continued with the session Scott spoke about how as I blossom it would also be nice to be able to be taken out for a coffee date, not even a meal, by a man. And bingo my stuff was up again.

I could not receive even a cup of coffee from a man.

I feel all my stuff in my physical body as it surfaces. As I have worked with Scott I am paying more attention to my body when something does not feel right, and not to override it.

My whole body on the left side started to contract and I started to feel like a mouse. The mouse wanted to leave the room and scurry into the forest. The mouse was running wild, frantically spinning in circles. I could not stay present, I was just freaking out to get out of there.

The mouse was hiding in its mouse house. It was like the mouse had something to share with me. I got my protector snake to act as a protector to the mouse so that the mouse could calm down. The snake circled the mouse and the mouse could start to relax in the space.

As the frantic energy of the mouse calmed down I could feel in my body where there were lines or tubes of spite. These tubes of spite had been fed to me. It seems when I am in these states I am seeing things that I have not seen before. It is as though there were tubes still feeding me the spite. My body was still being fed poison. This, by the way, is happening on an energy level; however it is definitely happening still on the physical level. And although chances are that those who fed me are long dead and gone, the energy lines are still open and still taking in this poison.

This is new for me, to be seeing how the poisonous energy lines from all past woundings were still active and alive.

The little girl believed she was only worthy of being fed poison and spite.

As I am learning boundaries I could feel into what a cup of coffee actually meant to me. Without boundaries I would take in anything, good or bad. It would mean that I would still be fed spite or poison and it was that which was upsetting me and my whole body. It was not the coffee but the learned acceptance of swallowing poison. I had learned it from a young age especially from my mother whose looks at me and silent disapproval I would swallow.

It was only when I was in my twenties that I finally heard how she spoke to me. We were on holiday in Israel and for the first time I heard her derogatory way of talking to me. It was an eye opener that it took so long to actually hear how she spoke to me. I guess it's protection, or survival. Trust me I have spoken to many in such a way.

In the session it felt as though there was a prickly sea creature that my hand was holding onto. Still accepting poison into my body. I was holding this creature with my left hand and it was still stinging me. I did not seem to want to let it go. Still holding onto the old way of being. It was great for me to be able to witness it and to see how the old patterns want to stay and I seem to want to hold onto them even though I know they are no good. I guess it is the pieces of a puzzle that fit together and until this puzzle changes it will continue. By doing this work I am changing my original beliefs on a cellular level.

I started to do some tapping work to release the belief that I deserve to be fed poison. It is interesting to look back at my previous eating habits which were certainly toxic. This whole journey began with my relationship to food yet has now bought up all things toxic in my system.

It was deep and intrinsic to the little girl to accept spite and poison. Eventually I called in the protector snake to help with shifting this and the snake formed a circle; I called all who had been spiteful to me to enter the circle. I then placed all spite that was fed to me at their feet.

As I kept doing this a sense of freedom started to enter.

With this release of all past toxins, the energy shooting through my body was so intense I had to lie down.

I felt my energy body become luminous green as though I had green wings and all around me was luminous energy. This energy filled the old toxic lines with new light and sealed the input lines of toxicity.

My true self had been weighted down by toxicity and now that it was given back to from where it came, I was shifting big time.

The energy was so expansive, way bigger than this body, touching all corners. Luminous green. As though I were a human butterfly.

I was totally high on this energy. I felt myself in Hawaii in the sacred temple of Akalani. I was in the centre of the temple and there were 28 sacred rocks around me. I was very big. These are the 28 energies I had brought through in 2010. I then experienced three other layers. It was as though those who had trained me in real life and spirit life were celebrating me. I was so expansive and so luminous. No way could I have sat upright at that point. It was the first time I saw Scott had provided a cushion for me to lie down on. He certainly was one step ahead of me. I was all the light, the luminous one.

I vibrated in this energy for a while and then I was given a ball of light to place in my heart and given the instruction to use this wisely. And this is the crux. I had been inappropriately giving it and rescuing everyone. It was now time to use it wisely.

My hands were pulsating luminous green light. My whole body was pulsating and vibrating and yet I could still communicate with Scott through it all. He then asked me to go to my other spiritual home, Table Mountain. My energy changed to more of a quieter light. And finally to come back to where I am now in Australia.

It is here where I can embody this. It is a safe place for me to embody it. I brought all that energy back into my body as I was aware that I had to get in a car and drive.

I was high as a kite, drunk on life, yet with my training with the Kahunas I was trained to change feet mid-air. I knew I would be safe to drive.

The beauty of being able to time travel without getting on an aeroplane in the time of Covid is amazing. And Scott gets to travel along as well. It is a total homecoming of all that I am.

I believed I was a fat, miserable, rich, poor child.

Trust me, that is so gone from every cell of my body.

I carried that which was placed on me by family friends and others for so, so long. It is not mine to carry. That is their stuff. I am a luminous being of light. I am freedom expressed in this body. I am fearless. I am creative. I am a celebration on two legs.

Things I learnt from Scott

His love in the kitchen was passed onto me.

Chapter 13: The Three Lands

How does one describe a shamanic session where I can be in three lands at once?

I have spent many years as a shamanic body worker and so I understand the body from seeing it above the body and seeing it in the body. The seeing part is not with the physical eyes but with the psychic eyes.

The body is the most awesome thing, especially when it comes to trauma. How it is able to encapsulate the trauma and when ready, reveal what it has held onto.

All the talk therapy is not likely to come close to what the body has stored.

My first experiences of the power of the body to hold the trauma safely locked away was through my training in Hawaiian massage.

It was during my first training whilst I was being massaged that I moved into the most primordial screaming session. The poor students at the time had no idea what to do with me and removed their hands from me.

At that session it felt as though I was stuck in the birth canal. Metaphorically what was happening was that the traumas in my body were starting to exit from their deep state of numbness. It was many years later that I got to remember what I had blocked.

I was so distraught after that session I sought out the Kahuna. A Kahuna is the Hawaiian master of his field. In this instance, my Kahuna was a master of the physical body and of course everything else related to it. He was able to put his hands on me and I physically felt my organs shifting. That was the first time I had felt such power from a person. I also got to experience the ability of seeing with my eyes closed in that training. Seeing through the ability of my hands and senses.

At that time I had no idea what I was unearthing from my body but it was the first step. I continued my training with the Kahuna for many years and it was as though he kept waiting for me to release these trapped memories.

Keep in mind that the body holds onto them until it is safe enough to release them. This is vital. Early unveiling of such traumatic memories could send one mad.

The first traumatic memory to be released was the motor accident. It has been years of work dealing with that.

The next layer of releasing was related to the abuse.

I have had different insights over the years but it is now whilst I am in therapy that all the pieces are coming together.

Today's session began with me saying how I am numb when I eat, I have the feeling I don't deserve to eat and food is holding no pleasure for me.

By this point I am a good cook so it's not about the food I am making.

I also expressed that I was feeling bloated like a poisonous fish.

Last week was the first time I witnessed the aftermath of being abused. It was the first time I got to see what happened to me after I was abused, with fish being thrown at me, and me discarded like a piece of meat.

I fully understand that had these memories emerged all at once, I most probably would have gone mad and so it is with deep reverence to the wisdom of the body that I share my story now.

I also told Scott that I was feeling bloated and fat like I had taken on the body form of the abuser. Never had I seen that before.

Working with Scott I am able to really embody and move my body whilst working with him. Allowing my body to move, hunching over, and stooping and twisting around. My body becomes contorted. It is in the moving of the body that the release of the stuck memories can start to shift.

This session began back with me in the hut where the abuser was holding me like a piece of meat, upside down, in his big hands. He was being sucked off by a woman. After he came he flung me to the floor. I was lifeless with blood on my body, unable to move and fish were being thrown at me. The bones and heads of fish.

I was lifeless and even unable to respond to

what Scott was suggesting.

I then saw a witch doctor in the room holding a bone and it was me being cursed as a White child. As though all their hatred and vulgarity was put on me.

I had the feeling that I deserved it. Logically the adult knew this was not right but I was so stuck there. Scott invited me to purge it into a bowl he had provided. It was as though the little girl was not willing to let it go. He did say to me it's what she has known and it is familiar.

It felt as though I was surrounded by a black spider over my full body and inside I had a pit of snakes in my stomach. Again I could not move it.

Scott invited me to start tapping my chest to move the energy. I was then able to get the black snakes inside of me moving. All snakes had beliefs attached to them. I am dirty, ugly, disgusting, not worthy.

The snakes were then eaten by my protector snake, bar the last one that was the abuser's one. This snake I could smash and kill against a rock. It was at this point that the little girl finally could get up and start to stab all the abusers in the room. I know from working as a therapist this way that this is the moment that energy can come back. Numbness is the state of shutdown. Movement is where the healing is able to begin.

She sliced and killed everyone. Except the nanny.

I got to see that not only had I taken on the

abuser's body shape but I was also carrying his whole tribes' anger, hatred and disgust.

No wonder my constant head talk was that I was fat/heavy. I was fat from all this crap I have been carrying. I knew always my weight had nothing to do with food. So few could hear me on that. Certainly no doctor. I was looked at as obese due to over-eating. Everyone would suggest a new diet. Yet I was hardly eating. It was this, this crap of others that I was carrying. The load of curses, tribal hatred, and vendettas that the Blacks were waging on the White children. I do know I am not alone in this form of abuse. What a big load for an innocent child to carry.

The little girl was then able to sit on a child chair and see the carnage in the hut. She had her energy back. She left the hut with myself as the adult, she as the child and the nanny whose hands were still tied and her head hanging low. And watched as the littel girl burnt the hut down. Now free.

The little girl was able to be in my arms now. Scott invited me to bath her. My immediate feeling was to take her to Hawaii, my spiritual home. But still it did not feel clear. In hindsight I see that the nanny could not enter Hawaii so the further work had to be done back in South Africa where the original abuse had happened.   I took the little girl back to Cape Town and this time to Table Mountain. She was happy for me to bath her in the streams of the rivers. Table Mountain is a majestic mountain with a flat table top and on either side, smaller peaked mountains. Often clouds spill over the top to the mountain like a table cloth.

The stream I took her to was pristine, flowing over rocks. Lush vegetation. She was in her element. However, I still had the nanny hanging around, with her heaviness. And even still I was wanting to look after her. I mean all this work and I want to look after the abuser. Scott directed me to give it all back to her. I was able to put all the abuse and guilt and shame and shit into sacks and load her up. She was covered in so many black sacks. I then sent her on her way in a carriage run by demons and cleared up the residue.

The little girl was in her element, free as a bird frolicking in the water. There were butterflies surrounding her, the trickling water and shimmering light. Bells were on her ankles. It was as though she was a fairy totally in her element. She was also able to communicate with the mountains and to understand the love of the mountain. In a way I feel as though she is a child of this mountain and the unwavering love of Table Mountain has been with her. It was as though she had come home to her true home, the mountain.

A lifetime of curses and possible more life times had been lifted. What a karma I must have come into this life with.

In her pure joy and delight I was able to also connect with Hawaii and to Mount Warning in Australia.

I was standing in three lands with the little girl in the middle in pure light and love. A triangle of powerful mountains and the little girl in the centre, dancing her light. Pure light, pure joy, pure innocence.

Hawaii is my spiritual home and I have very

strong former memories of past lives and the beauty of having received my training there this life time. I always feel that my knowledge from Hawaii was way deeper than this life time. Working as a shamanic body worker I often felt too young to know so much. I guess now that I am older it balances out.

Africa, my homeland where I experienced such savage and raw trauma is my home where I grew my resilience and the place where I now see that such darkness can be transformed into pure light.

Australia, the place that welcomed me with such open arms and acceptance. The place where the wisdom of the land is honoured by its custodians.

I got to see that this little girl knows lands. The adult had learned bodies. First from the Western way though university training and then through the shamanic way through the Hawaiian temple massage training.

From an early age she was tapped into lands and this is the reason why I have had magical and spiritual experiences with different lands including Greece and Lord Howe Island.

I am a living example of being gutsy enough to face such deep cruelty and darkness and to emerge into the light.

This step of the journey I know required someone to hold my hand due to the horrific nature of it.

And yes, I am the one who has had the courage to face it and emerge as light.

Now having experienced all that, I can fully release from all levels, the roles of the abusers and company, who played their part. I do not need any further abuse to awaken me to the light.

I am a light being born into purity, that purity was knocked so far out of me. I reclaim that purity now and am deeply grateful to the amazing masters, teachers and of course Scott.

Things I learnt from Scott

Get messy and tactile in the kitchen.

Chapter 14: Illness

Today I was reminded of the traits of my star sign. Capricorn. The achiever.

I am not one to know much about star signs but I know a bit about my Capricorn sign.

We are old when we are young. As a twenty-year old I was like an old lady, very conservative and conformist. Boring as all hell.

Now as a 66-year-old I want to be in nightclubs partying the night away. Granted night-clubs that are smoke free and alcohol free and for the unvaccinated. I love being around younger people - it energises me.

I was reminded that Capricorns love projects. This is so true of me, in fact all the men in my past whom I dated were my projects. I projected on them how they would be the famous dancers, teachers or film-makers. They became my full-time projects and I became obsessed with how they would be IT. So much energy and time going into each man. Not only putting energy into them but every second word out of my mouth was their name. Oh, how I cringe now.

I also of course undertook many other projects starting at a young age where I organized, together with a friend, a concert on an island as a fund raiser. I was only 15. Five thousand people attended that concert. I organised dental conferences and other fundraisers as well, and numerous art exhibitions and parties. I could pull off events at a drop of hat. I still can.

The only problem with someone like me is when the projects dry up.

It was usually on my return from my hedonistic lifestyle in Cape Town to Byron Bay that I felt a drought on the projects/lover side. In Cape Town I would tell men who desired me to get into the queue. I would be the queen of my domain. Byron Bay is awesome and a great town to be in. However, for me I am never met by men here, especially after experiencing black men in the true sense. Yes, once you go black you never come back...

This time in the drought here, the attention turned inward to me and the project became illness. More specifically my illness.

The shamans ask - when did you stop dancing and painting? So true of the journey I was just on.

In this last year I took that project of sickness on big time. Overnight my hands virtually became crippled. It was Christmas 2020. Suddenly it was painful even to drive. My whole body went into a painful state. Rolling over in bed was difficult.

The project then became doctors and X-rays and pathology tests. I was hobbling around like an old woman. Even though my age is up there I have never been an old woman. What with young lovers and nightclubs, that did not enter my reality.

I became depressed and miserable.

I felt friendless, miserable, in pain and could not see the purpose of living. This was the dark night of the soul for me. Second time round. I had also experienced that dark night round the age of thirty.

This time I had to go so deep and so low to pull out the hidden memories that were still troubling me.

Now I am on the other side of it. The gratitude to have a healthy body again is wonderful. There are no more body aches or pains. It took about 10 months to clear the body. I contribute this to a few things, including homeopathy.

I have a great homeopath who is in Cape Town who will work with me online. The Bowen therapy - I describe it as having the body cleared inside with a brush. Very subtle and profound.

And most importantly my kitchen therapy.

The project at this point, away from illness, is being creative again. This time in the writing and cooking. For some reason I have not wanted to paint at all in this period of my life. Painting used to be my biggest go-to to release my internal monsters.

Initially when I first started painting round the age of 25 I used to paint just monsters. Everything that had bottled up inside me came out in the paintings. As I became happier in life the paintings shifted until the last time I painted it was of happy dancers in bright colours.

In South Africa I was dancing the most seductive dance called Kizomba. I used to paint dancers both on their bodies and on canvas and do live art demonstrations where I would whip up a painting in two songs and then get to dance with the teacher. That was the highlight of the night.

It was when I came back to Australia, with no Kizomba dancing and no lovers that I believe I started to play with illness.

And play with it I did.

I forgot about my love of dancing: for me it is a love language without words. An intimate journey of two people together. Meeting in energy bliss.

The writing that follows was written five years ago and is still relevant today.

The Dance of the beloved.

I am going to share my story of dancing. From my earliest recalls until today my belief was that I was just plain and simply fat. Not beautiful, not intelligent, not capable. JUST FAT.

It feels that this is such a waste of a precious life to have such deep negative beliefs of myself. Where did such a belief begin? I would imagine from early childhood abuse and from a mother who was obsessed with her body perfection and her inability to love this wild child.

Dancing was a foreign concept to me until after my divorce when I began to explore different modalities and it was always the difficulty of letting a man lead me. Although I remained fat throughout the years despite dancing, it was whilst dancing that I felt liberated.

I persevered in learning Salsa and remained constantly on the level of "Blah" dancer despite paying my teachers enough to put their kids through college.

No offense to the teachers, maybe I was just a bad student. I reached the point with Salsa where now, even the music irritates me. So, to all the men who never asked me to dance, no need now, I am over Salsa.

Four years ago, I came across the music and dance called Kizomba. This was an instant love affair. Finally, I had found a dance that satisfied my wild sensual self, music that I loved and an embrace that made me bloom.

I also soon realized that the western way of adapting the dance was not satisfying at all. I started a quest to find an Angolan dance teacher.

I found an Angolan restaurant, Praia Morena, in Cape Town, and persuaded the owner to have Kizomba nights. It was there I met Davide and in that moment I knew I had found my teacher.

It took me three years of asking him to please teach me that he finally agreed. (Maybe he hesitated because he knew he was about to face his most difficult student.) Luckily my passion overtakes my inability as a dance student.

Davide was born to dance. Whichever partner he dances with, he makes them feel like a million dollars. Although I was dancing with him for those first three years and believing I was amazing dancing with him, I have come to understand he adapts to make his partner look good. He can do this with everyone.

When our lessons began the first thing that came up was that I actually had no idea how to dance this dance. Now to everyone looking at this dance it does not look that complicated, but to me here, this fat 61-year-old, it certainly brought up my issues. There were many a times when he was on the floor coaxing my legs into position. Despite that, my love of dancing and especially the love of Kizomba will continue regardless of age, size, or physical challenge.

And it is not only dancing that this remarkable man is teaching - it is about life. There have been two very pivotal moments in the dance that have rocked me and changed me. One was when he told me I was not willing to learn, all I wanted to do was to dance. Eek, that was really true, but if I wished to dance with other Angolan men then I was going to have to pull it in and learn the real way.

The other moment was when he told me I could not trust him, in the dance. And in that moment, I saw it was in life that I could not trust a man to support me.

It is not just dance lessons I am in the process of with this remarkable man but life lessons.

His timing in confronting me in such a loving way was when I was able to go the deepest with myself and see my own patterns.

I have watched Davide operate for four years now. And I only see love. He has been attacked and betrayed by other teachers in town and he remains calm and in love. Such a lesson for me, this reactive wild woman, to witness.

I have seen him dance with 75-year-olds, with women fatter than me, with a woman in a wheel chair, and all of them are so deeply touched.

He makes everyone feel loved. He brings the best out in his students, both male and female.

The world would be a better place if there were more Davide's as dance teachers.

A blessing to this life to have met such a young remarkable man and I will be there to see him rise to such fame.

He was one of my projects that I have had to walk away from. I was spoilt in that dance connection and I do not know if I will ever feel that connection again on the dance floor.

Things I learnt from Scott

Have no judgment when sugar cravings take over.

Chapter 15: The cook, nanny and garden boy

23 November 2021

Today's session might be the hardest one to capture.

I arrived today, really well, in full positive energy and ready to look at what my discomfort was still with my childhood family home.

At this point once again I thought: I have looked at the worst so this should be a breeze. Little was I to know what would surface.

All the sessions are approached in full trust that Scott can get me through it and I aim not to be the therapist. I mean after all, as a therapist I should have sorted all this out by now.

So regressing back to the age of about four, I entered my home. It was a sterile place for me. Each room was like a mausoleum. Cold, hard and bitter were words I used. There was no room I felt comfortable in. And the kitchen was an area I was banned from as it was the nanny and the cook's domain. There was no recollection of me being able to go to a fridge and even help myself to an apple. I wondered how I was fed at all. The place was sterile and hostile to me. My room was devoid of toys. However, my brother's room had aeroplanes and more life in it.

Scott asked where I could go to be safe, but it felt that there was no safe space for me. I felt that I could try and hide in the corner of my room. There was no human I could connect with and the only connection I had was to my dog Rusty. That was the only love I felt. My brother and I fought all day.

I felt such disdain towards me from everyone in that household. Nowhere was welcoming to me.

I felt in my body that there was a weight on my shoulders and when we looked further I was still carrying the guilt of the motor accident. Guilt given to me by both my parents and the deceased nanny. I was able to return this guilt once again to their feet. I saw how I had been the scapegoat of the family, carrying this weight for all of them. As I went into a circle, all of them were yapping at my feet. I looked at all their facades and saw such ugliness behind the good-looking masks of my parents and all in the room. I had taken on and was carrying their ugliness. I was able to get into my power and destroy most of the house except the kitchen.

I was able to return it all and get my light back. At this point I was happy to lie down on the magic cushion and go to spiritual wonderland.

Basically, a spiritual bypass was what I wanted. This is common in the spiritual community. Off to fairyland without doing the work.

However, my body was presenting more stuff to be looked at.

In these sessions my body goes into real pain to show me where I am holding stuck information. I know Scott can see it as well as he invited me not to lie down and to see what else was in the body.

It felt like there was a skewer through my left

shoulder blade affecting my heart as well. Both shoulders were tensed up. I said I feel like a piece of meat whose shoulder had been hacked off.

My heart felt like a solid black mass and I was feeling physical pain in it.

I felt hands on my shoulders and got the insight that I had been lifted by one arm, pulling my shoulder out.

I returned to the kitchen and there was a stand-off between the cook, the nanny and the garden boy.

They would not look at me. They saw me as a rich white bitch who had red hair who was the devil incarnate. There could be superstitions around red-haired people, who knows. My hair was not just red, it was bright auburn red.

They could not look me in the eye. Ever.

Keeping in mind these are the people who were paid to feed and care for me.

I felt this hand on my shoulder, a big hand that would not let go.

Scott invited in all the hands who were holding me. There were many.

It felt like the nanny was wanting something from me.

I tuned in, the first word that came was money.

Yet she would not let go.

There was a tug of war between her and the

garden boy.

At this point I freaked out in the session as I saw I had been the bait that was used between them. I asked Scott to hold my hand as I could feel me about to slip into something dark and I wanted to feel a link to this world. Hell had arrived. I started to scream and hyperventilate. Sobbing raw sobs. I was back in the maid's room where I was being physically abused.

She had used me as bait, feeding me to the garden boy, so he could carry out abuse on me. Money was exchanged for this.

I saw myself in the maid's room, the top half of me was being burnt by cigarettes, I could not feel my lower half but I could see blood. I could see him with his erection. It was too intense on my body reliving this so I floated above my body. Many hands and cocks were inserted into me and they burned the inside of my vagina with cigarettes. I could smell the burning of my flesh. I could smell the semen. There were many people there in the maid's room at my childhood home. No wonder it was not a place of warmth.

I was once again discarded in the corner whilst they all partied. The question is where were my parents and again I imagine that they were out and I was left in the maid's care.

This scene was horrific for me to see today. It is devastating to see how much abuse was dished out onto me.

And it had been in a 60-year memory vault only to be opened today. It is as I get stronger in myself that I can see this and be able to bring it to some form of closure or peace. I fully get why the vault had been sealed for so long. I also get why I had to let go of most people at this time as the panacea to pretend all is well is over.

It is not. My body has been through horrific unknown episodes of cruelty and abuse. By those who were paid to love me. Whilst my own parents could not love me.

It is a major shock on my system to see all this and I also know the value of using compost to grow flowers.

I have survived such horrific abuse and I am writing about it. The reason I write is that it is purged out of my body: this a farewell to all the abuse that this body has experienced.

I am not surprised I have carried weight all my life. The weight of other's ugliness. The weight of the imbalances in a skewered country. The weight of terror. The weight of being the scapegoat. The weight of being feared as the devil. The weight of being feared for my light. The weight of the abuse.

And I wonder at this point - did my Kahuna teachers see all this that I was carrying? Did Papaji know as well?

I had no idea it was that ugly and that deep.

It has been seen now and so it is a resurfacing of myself, having seen all that, to find that strength in me again.

I write this book so that none of this will spill out onto my children or grandchildren as I more than anyone know that what is not healed will be played out and usually by later generations.

I lay in the corner of that room. In fact, part of me has been laying there all this time. My little girl would not come to me. She did not trust even me. And why should she as I had also pushed her away and out of sight from me?

I did apologise to her and managed to get her back to me and to the safe space of Table Mountain.

I then experienced myself in Hawaii at the temple where I shared the words that the test of a Kahuna is to swim with the sharks.

They would either die or become a Kahuna.

My testing began at a very young age and now I know for sure I have swum with many sharks.

I have survived.

To my little girl I am so, so sorry that you had to go through so much hard abuse and be left so alone in it. I did not know that this had happened until today. And even in seeing it I wanted to run away, going no, this can't be true. However, it is being witnessed as true through both my body and Scott seeing it as well. It is true and I am so, so sorry you had to go through that. I would not wish that on my worst enemy. And how you survived it blows my mind. I don't know how you survived it. You must be one incredible child to survive such horrors.

It is almost like you are the carrier of the horrors of apartheid. As though you were the Joan of Arc carrying all this stuff. I know you lost your voice a long time ago about this but now as you heal and feel me with you, I am so curious about how you survived it.

The adult heart is open now and I would love it if you could tell me your side of this story from your perspective. *I believed it was my fault and needed to take the punishment.*

How come you believed that? *They kept telling me I was the devil's child.*

When it happened did you cry? *No, I took it. I whimpered.*

Why did you not tell your parents? *They would not believe me.*

How often did it happen? *Often. Weekly on a Saturday when they went out.*

How did your parents not see your burn marks? *They never bathed me.*

I still smell the burning flesh.

Let's let the water of Table Mountain heal it. For now. I believe you.

No one ever believed me.

My flesh is still burning and I still smell it. Ok little one I believe you fully. I will use Akalani 13 to help bath you. And take away the smells. *The smells are stuck in my throat.* I hear you little one, I believe you.

I want to vomit. Can I hold you to try to vomit it

out? Ok.

I feel so shattered now.

I wonder how anyone gets through such horrific abuse?

I am in tears at this point and they are long-stored tears that need to be released. My body is shaking and just sadness now is present.

I do know if I can't get through this, Scott will be there, so I will continue. I want to be held as a child now. To be cared for. Something I do not know.

And on the flip side I know I have had major training in trauma release throughout all my body work training.

For my little girl now I am as devastated as you are. Let's both just cry in the waters of Table Mountain. For the loss of my childhood. For the loss of what feels like my life. For the loss of innocence, for the abuse of all in South Africa. And I, as a child, cannot carry that abuse for South Africa or anyone any more. I put that abuse at your feet South Africa. I am a child and to carry that is too much even for me as the adult.

So I hold my little one now and I will speak to you South Africa. I have carried that guilt, that shame, that hurt, that abuse for all these years and I cannot nor will I carry it another day further. I put all the abuse of the black/white story at your feet, Table Mountain. It is not for me to carry it. I have carried it for too long.

And I allow you now to speak through me, South Africa.

Speak to me of your abuse without me being the carrier of it. Speak to me that I may hear you without judgment.

It has no voice as yet.

Is there a voice of abuse that wants to talk to me?

Yes.

It was a Maya (illusion) that one day you would let go of the importance of carrying all this weight. It made you feel important carrying it. You felt special carrying such a weight, like a Joan of Arc, like a chosen one.

Did I feel I was healing the world? *No.*

Now it is a triumphant moment as I walk through the abuse, allowing my body now to receive healing from the mountain, allowing my womb to be washed. And now allowing the true mommas of Africa to hold me again. Those who are loving. And loving they do know. In Me going with African men later in life was me wanting this, the being held by Africa. The loving Africa, not the abusive one.

I will also rest this body at the ubuntu (peace) tree which will soothe my spirit.

My body healing is in the waters of Table Mountain. My spirit shock to be healed by the ubuntu tree.

This tree I met just before I left South Africa last time. It holds a lot of magic and is at the foot of Table Mountain which is recognised as the seventh natural wonder of the world. When I met this tree, I was so knocked out by its energy that I had to lie there for hours. It is so strong with people who know it. There is a story of a Kenyan man who walked all the way from Kenya to meet the tree. It knows me as well.

And so now as I sit in Australia I allow the spirit of South Africa's true essence to heal me.

And what is South Africa for me? It is passion, it is life, it is dance, it is rhythm, it is colour. It throbs – it is a living force.

Things I learnt from Scott

A plate of food can be a work of art.

Chapter 16: Sad and shattered

25 November 2021 (morning)

Scott

There is a tendency to want to protect you from this, my heavy story.

I know you especially don't need protection and I want to honour you - you must have done some of your own heavy lifting to stand by me on this journey.

I am still crying and I will not stop the tears from flowing.

It helps me to know that you are there as I touch such a depth of abuse and depravity that was spewed onto this body.

That I could only feel like a piece of meat and not like a human being.

The image of a shoulder of lamb still lingers in me. That is how my own shoulder felt when I was being dragged by the nannies.

I am still so saddened by such depravity that was dished out onto me.

I have not told you much about what it was like growing up in an apartheid society.

Most white families acted like they were superior, with at least two servants on call all the time.

There was an arrogance from the whites towards the blacks. The blacks were regarded as second-class citizens. Slaves most probably would be a better term to use.

With the end of apartheid this attitude actually still exists. Many looked down on me for dating black men. Looked at me like I was less than them, that I couldn't date a white man. There is a spirit in me which, despite all that has happened, also knows the black spirit, the passion and the strength.

Apartheid tried to kill the soul of the black people. It could not. Their spirit is so strong.

They were kept menial, in education, in work, in life. Living in shanty towns, not able to board the same bus as white people. Not able to go to cinemas or beaches.

How they did not rise up and slaughter the whites I don't know. Then again, they were revenge-abusing the kids, and I was one of them.

The women were separated from their own families to look after the white peoples' children. Not getting time to spend with their own children. Their grannies would bring up their children whilst they worked for menial pay.

I too as an adult followed this way of life. I had two servants and on their days off I would go to pieces as to how could I cope?

I could not cook or clean. I had people pick up my dirty clothes off the floor. Embarrassing but this was true.

I had dreams for many years after I left South Africa that I had forgotten to pay the maids. Also the garden boy. Eventually I set up an automatic payment system in my dream world so they would be paid. I left the garden boy's payment to my husband. Interesting that those dreams still lingered of the garden boy. Now I know why.

It is interesting the term garden "boy", not even man. Again, the diminishing of people.

I did get to spend time in townships later in life as a visitor and I could see the warmth that existed within the townships and the constant welcoming between neighbours. There was a buzz in the townships despite the poverty.

This is a very sick society to grow up in where superiority is reigned upon others. It still exists.

I used to say South Africa was honest in the fact that it openly declared its racial views. Not nice but true. Most other countries are racists without admitting it.

I was shocked when I arrived in Australia that there was apartheid here, even though unspoken. And that same superiority is now dished out onto the First Nations people with the current genocide through the vaccine. I was shocked by the stolen children story.

I was naive in believing that only South Africa practised apartheid. That naivety did not last long.

Apartheid is segregation to assume superiority. Divided outside yet that division is inside as well. Afraid of that which is different to you.

Black has been labelled "the bad". The black people carry this load.

And the confusion for a white child to be brought up by a black person who is belittled and hated by her own parents. How sick! How sick is the whole world now as well?

Evening writing

Scott I am finding that I am wanting to protect you from my story and not even come or call again.

It's like I can't believe anyone can care for me. But I will stick to the course.

I am fragile as all shit.

I manage to function in the day and now in the evening let myself cry it out.

I could go to dancing and pretend all is well. It is not well and I need to not run away from it.

Camping is off for now and that's maybe a good thing so I can be in the safe space of my home and cry when I need to.

I am still however managing to eat well. I do have lots of prepared meals.

What would I want in this phase of my life? To be held and cry uncontrollably for days – it's not going to happen but I can at least let the tears flow when I write.

So much built up grief.

For now, it is most probably better that I just grieve alone.

I am shattered.

I am in pieces, I am hurting.

And it worries me that I even want to run from you.

Because I do trust you and know you are there for me in a professional sense.

My heart is broken that so much bad stuff happened to me.

I have no idea how the little girl survived it.

Interestingly my back has pock marks that I thought was from acne and also I had a cancer removed from my back. These must be the scars from the cigarette burns.

Writing does help me and also that I am writing to someone.

I cannot face a paint brush.

I can't face people now.

I am just sad, sad, sad.

I will let this sadness play its course.

Not to run to chocolates or dancing, just to be sad. Heart-broken. And allow it to be.

I know we are not given more than we can cope with. But for now it hurts. My heart is shattered. Can I ever recover and trust people?

I also know I have had strong training but for

now I need to just grieve. A life that was created from abuse.

A life of no love. I do however know I love my kids and grandkids so I am capable of love.

I do know my granny loved me.

26 November 2021

Shattered.

Scott. I still feel I want to protect you from my horrid story even now in the writing of it. But I won't.

Is it shame that makes me want to hide it all now, even from you?

I still am shattered.

My little girl is not at the mountain, she is hovering above.

I fear also that her hands were tied. It feels that that memory is in my body too.

And the feeling of this is too much for me to handle; death would be easier.

I don't know how I survived it.

I don't know how I will survive this. But yes, I am a fighter so I will get through it. Maybe the biggest fight of my life is to survive this now.

Of all my memories of accidents, rapes etc this feels the hardest to deal with.

The fact it was hidden from me for so long.

That I had no idea. There were dreams of that room though. Uncomfortable feelings in my dreams.

And yes, my hands have been tied. I feel it especially in my left hand.

This whole journey of the original so-called illness started with suddenly painful hands.

At the time I thought it was past life memory of me being dragged behind a horse. Do I put things in past life memory when it is too hard to deal with in this life?

The little girl is suspended in the air. She can't get to the mountain where she frolics. She can't frolic now, she is frozen above.

I am so shattered. And yes, it is far safer for me to be home now, not camping. At least my home is beautiful and protective for me now. I have had blinds put up which makes it more private and safer for me to weep alone here. My tendency in the past was to go off to holiday in a different country, anything to just keep moving. Evidently away from what I had to face.

It also feels safe for me to have someone on the property as well. At least there is another human close by.

I did some random writing previously to all about this: my brother could not hear it, my father did not believe it, my mother could not give a shit. My grandmother wanted to kill.

It is all the loneliness in dealing with such a story.

In that writing were friends from the past:

Steven and Mush were there for me. And Mush's mum believed me.

Growing up, Mush was where I went to for some warmth in a house. Her mum used to feed me biscuits. In later life I did spend time with her mum who really liked me.

It was the so not being accepted by my own family - no fucken' warmth at all, no fucken' chocolate or biscuit given to me.

So I sit with this trauma, with no basis of love to feel support in the horror of it. Not even energetically can I get support from my own family. Still dead, cold and gone.

And my living brothers, no chance of support at all.

Possibly my cousin could give me support but I can't talk to him now. I can't talk to anyone now.

I have created aloneness in this trauma. I was alone then and I am alone now.

Somehow, I have to try get the little girl back.

I do know we have walked through stuff and eventually I will walk through this. At this point it feels too much for me.

It is too much. It is too much for a human to survive that.

I must be one hell of a human to have survived that.

And yes, I imagine there is a reason for it but at this point I am just in the aftermath of being shattered.

I won't fight that. These tears are well overdue. I cry for the loss of innocence. I cry for a little girl who was so abused and survived it. I cry for having no-one I can trust to support me. I cry for myself.

I cry for my little girl who is so shocked out of existence.

Will my tears ever stop? I don't know. But I do know I can still function and finish dealing with builders. (Tomorrow is the last day for this final renovation.)

There is this amazingly powerful woman who can do things and a totally shattered and destroyed little girl. I am amazed at my own tenacity to get things done, even now whilst shattered.

See you Tuesday.

Things I learnt from Scott

Drop all old diet /starve concepts. Find true nourishment.

Chapter 17: How?

Hi Scott it is now 4 days since the uncovering of the horrors.

I have stopped crying. I looked at myself today and do see that something has been cracked open.

I know there are still images trapped that need to be worked through but I will wait to work it with you as I know it is too big for me to handle alone. Burning flesh, hands trussed like a pig. Smells.

It was interesting to see that I wanted to run away even from you who is helping me. It is the "pack my bags and leave scene".

I did not run away to go camping, I have not run away from you. And I will spend the morning with my friend Shine. She is soothing for me. Her late partner was South African and I feel that he is the connection we have again. I feel him also supporting me in this horror.

I do know my resilience will get me through it and there must be a reason for it. I had an inkling of my hands being activated to something new. It is too soon to see what the new is and I will not rush it. I want all these horrors removed from my physical body.

And in this I think is it better to know what happened than to live in oblivion. The pain of the emotional side was so intense in this time. But I would rather it was out than in me. And yes, without a doubt, had this not been cleared, physical illness would have been the next step. In it I thought physical pain is better than this emotional pain. I let those thoughts go now.

I also had an insight: with the black men I dated I always felt like I owed them money. It is linked to that scene that I feel I am the payment.

I wonder how it has affected me in life? For one, not letting people close to me. Connecting stronger to spirit world than the real world. Not allowing love in on all levels. Being tough - I can do it myself. And of course, suppressing it all with food. I can now also see how, as the trauma was emerging closer to the surface, the desire for sugar increased.

Amazingly enough, through all of this in these last few days, I am cooking and feeding myself well. It was like I was being prepped for it - at least on the physical level I could take care of myself.

Writing has been a great source of comfort for me, either writing coherently or random writing which gets deleted straight away. Also to know I am writing to you has helped a lot and I do not hold back.

The questions still exist. How did I survive that?

How can I heal? How can I love? How could my parents not know? Mainly, how did she survive? What did she think, that it was her fault? So she took it.

This has been very, very intense for me to face and now to deal with.

I have had masters and Kahunas' in my life so that gives me some hope.

I also know that we touched such light in me before this came out as though it too was preparing me. And that light, how do I feel it now? It's there but with a cloud in between and that cloud I will face with you. It is too intense to face it alone now. Back then I had no one to help me through it, now I have you and I thank you.

I also know you can cope and it is not for me to worry about the amount of stuff I bring forward. It was interesting to see how I wanted to protect you. Who was I actually wanting to protect? I do not know.

I will see you on Tuesday. Thanks for being there for me. I will get through it.

Things I learnt from Scott

Tune into the body, what is it wanting.

Chapter 18: The missing piece of the puzzle

23 November 2021

Just before arriving for my session today, I received a reminder that 9 years ago on this day magic had happened. I was in Hawaii camping at a special beach spot and I had befriended a lady. She knew I was afraid of the ocean and somehow spent time with me to be brave enough to go deeper into the ocean. I guess this book has been exactly the same as that time. She took my hand and took me to the deeper waters. Scott took my hand and led me to the depths of where I had been afraid to go.

As I was swimming out into the ocean this time, on my own, a turtle swam under me. It led me further out than I had ever been. It stayed with me the whole way to the middle of the bay. As I lay on the surface of the ocean about 50 dolphins circled me. It was a remarkable experience and still lives with me today. It was a very high spiritual moment for me that could be described as pure love and grace.

I entered today's session grey, pale and trembling. After a week from hell of crying and wanting to take a one way walk into the ocean, I felt shaky walking into today's session.

I felt like I must have felt being dragged into the room to be abused. Yet the adult in me knew that there is total trust with Scott and I could get through it.

He asked what was still troubling me from uncovering those memories. I saw my little girl was still floating in fear. She had memories of blood, burning flesh, sperm and shit.

We had established that the abuse in the hut with the fish was prior to the abuse at home. The home abuse was an ongoing one. It was repeated and I imagine after each abuse, the memory was locked away. That locking away was what kept me sane in life.

The session started with me feeling into my stomach something that felt like a big black mass, like a wobbly Michelin man that was firmly in my stomach. There was a feeling like it was mine and for me to hold onto it. I was even ashamed to show it to Scott so firmly was I holding on to this black mass.

It was interesting that I wanted to continue to hold this mass. That I am strong enough to hold it plus the belief that I deserve to hold it. That I deserved all the abuse.

Somehow, I was able to manage to get it out of me, to be at a distance from me.

The little girl was afraid, in the corner, and she would not allow me to come close. I could get Scott in between her and the mass. He suggested that he took the position of watching the door and that I bring in an aspect of myself to help her feel safe. It was the protector snake.

The snake wrapped itself kindly around the little girl and the snake started to bring out the ugliness in my stomach. It was guilt mainly. It seemed like I had carried the guilt of the South African story forever. It was hard for me to release that one. I had to take myself off to Hawaii where I could do a release session. Feeding that guilt to the Hawaiian volcanoes. It seems I am able to do different releases in different lands as needed.

I could go back to the abuse room and saw that I carried revulsion, disgust, ugliness, sperm and hatred all in my body. With the help of the snake I was able to vomit over all the people in the room. There were lots of people in the room including one ring leader who was not the garden boy. I vomited over them all those qualities that they had put on me. I could see them drowning in what I had vomited on top of them. I could see how what they had put on me had stifled even my own breathing. I returned to them from whence it came that which was placed on me.

There was still a strong sensation in my throat. It felt like I was being choked. It felt as though sperm was drowning me.

I then had to face the garden boy. He was in a corner and at that point I felt like there were meat hooks in both my shoulders as though I had been skewered. This, was very painful in my body. I managed to return the meat hooks to him and skewered him with the hook. However, I could see he still had a chord attached to me, feeding all the crap into me. Into my womb. It is the same energetic tubes I had seen in previous sessions of me still being fed poison. Although the people are well dead and gone the poison energy was active and still being fed to me through energetic tubes.

I seemed to want to understand why I had the chord connection still. Scott suggested just to cut that chord. As soon as I cut it I felt like I had to birth a dead baby. I saw me giving birth to a dead baby and then all these creatures came running out of me.

Once all the creatures were out of me I felt that I needed a First Nations aunty to help me heal the womb.

I had met the Aunty about 20 years ago on a sacred trip to Uluru. I had been called via dreams to go to Uluru and had met up with seven other 'sisters' by coincidence. We were invited to a sacred healing ceremony. A rare invitation for Westerners. This was a healing gathering of First Nations people. At that time, we could not speak each other's language but the Aunty kept giving me the thumbs up.

She was back with me now to help heal my womb. I invited her into my womb where she brought the earth herbs to heal my womb.

I then saw myself on Ayers Rock with the aunties around me. I was surrounded by aunties. I was smudged and a ceremony was done for me. At the same time, I could feel my Hawaiian and African supporters there as well, as though three healing circles were happening at once.

The work was done on my womb and I felt myself back in Scott's house.

It was as though I had to undergo three different ceremonies in reclaiming myself. The healed version of me. A renovation of all that I had carried to the new version of me. The one who is not guilty, who does not carry shame, who does not carry others' baggage, who refuses to carry others' ugliness.

By the way, this journey was happening over the last 8 months whilst I was renovating a few different spaces in my house as well. Talk about reflecting the inside and outside.

This was the last version that needed to happen in Australia. The last piece of the puzzle.

My womb felt like it had become a triangle of light.

This time, rather than the pulsing green lights of fluorescent light, this was a golden light. A solid triangle of light that could vibrate at any speed. Much quieter and more solid.

My little girl, I would say for the first time, was so happy to lay upon me. She was so pure and so light. She was so proud of me as though she knew one day I could hold her again. Until now she could play away from me but never on me or with me.

That day has finally arrived. After all the dark evil shit that was put onto me I was able to return it to those who had dished it out on to me. It was no longer mine to carry.

I also met my mum and dad whilst I was clearing all the stuff. My mum was still cold. My dad was confused and on an energy level it came out that he did not know. Had he known he would have killed them all. Had he known he would have protected me. He sobbed many tears and he hugged me. He also brought in family who could believe me and to circle me and to offer protection finally. We were together in Hawaii with the dolphins around us.

On an energy level it at least felt like some form of human protection was being offered even though somewhat late. But for me it was a connection and most probably the connection that I could finally make with my little girl to actually feel her coming back to me.

I felt my womb light up and light Australia up, it lit up Africa and a deep gold light lit up Hawaii.

This energy was a golden light. If these energies had a smell I would be able to smell the gold, I would be able to smell the white light. I would be able to smell frangipani, from Hawaii. Blue Lotus in Australia and coconut from Africa.

These are my pure scents now. Nothing remains of the old scents.

These are the three lands that are vital to me. Africa my birthplace, the place I first experienced abuse. Hawaii my spiritual home, the place I remember my gifts from previous lives, and Australia, my safe haven now. The land of the indigenous that holds so much wisdom. The land that has now helped me heal a sick womb. These countries are firmly in my being and knowing them on a cellular level, I can travel energetically between them all and am welcome.

A useful skill to have in the time of Covid.

What had happened is past. It is now I am able to touch such light and embody it, bring in the smells and honour all that I am and all that I have been through. I am one hell of a survivor. I am a light warrioress, if such a word exists. I have walked through the darkness fully to claim my light now. To claim the roots of my Hebrew name. Leeorah. My light.

People I meet now I would like that they too have done the hard work. That they too vibrate on my level. Trust me this was no walk in the park. I will meet in pure light, I will meet others with a sweet strength, I will be met fully. It is also a time where I cannot hang onto old friendships that served me in the past to play the guilt and shaming trips. I have walked past that and if it means I have only one true friend left, so be it.

I thank you Shine for your grace to just hear me in my story and just to be there. To always be truthful and honest and always in such grace. I am so glad you are back in my life. I too feel David, your late partner, has my back too and has brought us together.

I deeply thank you Scott for having the courage to walk with me in this minefield, to come out the other side of it.

Finally to my little girl. Wow, I bow down to your strength. I bow down to your exuberance. I bow down to your amazing light and joy and purity. You are one hell of a kid and I am so pleased you can finally be back with me.

Welcome back.

Things I learnt from Scott

Accepting me warts and all.

Chapter 19: The body holds the score

My whole story is based around the effect of blocked memories.

As a bodyworker, with clients I was aware that the body was holding the memories in the subconscious memory bank. I never doubted what the body would present as it was more accurate than what the mind would divulge.

Working as a therapist, I was able to somehow read the body through the use of my hands, my closed eyes and my own body as a barometer. I was able to "see" inside the body on an energy level. I never doubted what was presented to me. However, it was not for me to tell the client what I saw. They had to experience it for themselves and I was well aware that certain information was not in their conscious minds.

I was able to tap into the subconscious belief patterns from their own lives and even their ancestors' lives. I had techniques that could shift these beliefs.

I had learned from my own experience in receiving this kind of bodywork that I too had blocked memories that were affecting my life.

The body will not release these memories until such a time that support systems are in place or that some form of balance is achieved.

From my own journey of the stored/blocked memories coming to the surface, there was a time lapse from the initial release to the uncovering of the memories.

It is like the body has a safety valve.

And very wisely so.

My initial blocked memories, when they surfaced, sent me into a spin and took many years to come to some sort of balance. In truth I believed I had uncovered all blocked memories.

I have to also give credit to the fact that because I had had these traumas I was able to stand by clients who were releasing traumas. I had the confidence that they would get through it.

Most clients would only need to see me once for a two-hour session.

In my case there was an inkling that all was not well. Despite the fact I thought I was so balanced. I mean after all, I was a dental hygienist and even lecturing to dentists.

I kind of started to suspect something was wrong when I first took up painting.

I began painting for the first time in my late twenties. I had never painted before, as that was my mother's domain.

The first painting I ever did was a very large oil painting. It was of four deeply traumatised faces.

It was at that point I thought, wow there might just be something wrong with me.

The first surfacing of blocked memories for me was 30 years to the day of the motor accident.

It blows my mind that the body could release them on the exact date. The body holds the score.

The body holds huge intelligence.

With the surfacing of those memories I did go to a therapist and I knew I needed support to make sense of these memories.

At that stage, when I was in my thirties, more memories did arise.

I was totally convinced that I had exposed all hidden memories and it was just a matter of balancing them.

The fact that I was left with the food/ kitchen stress should have alerted me to the fact that all was not well.

But as a "just do it" kind of a woman, life went on.

Life went on well. I was travelling the world. Working in Europe. Playing in South Africa and resting in Australia. I had it all down to a fine art.

My play time in South Africa was particularly fulfilling. I had my own art / dance studio where I could produce all the art I wanted to. I am prolific when that energy is on. Painting a 2 metre by 2 metre canvas in less than two hours. Once I was on a role I could whip up 5 paintings at a time. My best paintings are actually my fastest paintings.

And then, to host the best parties in town.

I was the queen of the Angolan community and my parties were renowned.

On the first Thursday of the month there would be art showings throughout the city. I was living in the city centre and was well placed for such an event.

I decided to open my art gallery on a whim, as I do. In less than 6 hours I produced numerous paintings, hung an exhibition and opened the same night. I sold a painting immediately. This painting could have been sold five times over. (I never understood what was seen in that painting!) I sold again at the next exhibition. And then, from there on, it just became a party place.

I would do live art sessions at these parties. I would paint my dance teacher dancing. In the duration of 2 songs I would have created a great painting. I would then get to dance with him albeit covered in paint. I gather you get it I am a messy painter. There certainly are no holds barred when I am painting.

As I am not a trained artist I don't have any restrictions on me, and this is where I believe my talent lies.

I was "in the zone" and even though there could be 40 people watching me I was unaware of them. It was me and the dancers and my canvas. It was as though I had entered another dimension.

An exciting opening was when I body painted my lover as part of the exhibition piece. It was the most erotic experience for both of us. The night progressed into dancing with a few of the models who had also been painted. These events were memorable.

My life really was a fairy tale. At a whim I could fly off to any country and satisfy any need.

Africa certainly was where I satisfied many a

need.

It is my birth country and once an African, always an African.

It is a river that flows in my blood. It is a river of passion, of wildness, of unbridled life that flows through me. I would be in conflict when I returned to Australia, to pull in all that passion. Hard to do after so much wildness and freedom.

By the way, I am different to most white South Africans, if you haven't gathered that yet.

South Africa is a land of such contrasts yet contains such a deep passion.

As I have had to go through the unveiling of my blocked memories, the passion still flows through my blood.

I have had to go through hell unblocking traumatic events that happened over 60 years ago. A hell that was covered up. Those memories were firmly stored in the safety of a memory vault, never to be opened until I had the support to get through it. Without that support I could have ended my life or gone mad.

That happened on the soil of my birth land.

Such deep trauma and abuse and yet I rise again. I believe at the time of the trauma I would have had to leave my body and be with the angels. It would have been the only way to survive. My early angelic training in life.

I rise again, clearer, having released that very heavy baggage.

I rise again knowing I have an incredible strength.

I rise again now knowing that playful, wild, passionate one in me is still alive. Despite what was put on me. It is not me. I am far greater than the shit that landed on me.

I rise again knowing that that incredible light I experienced after releasing the trauma is who I am.

I rise again knowing if I can get through this so can many.

I rise as a warrior woman. Deeply supported by the unseen guardians.

I rise again as woman unbridled.

I rise as the untold stories of many.

I rise as the light.

I rise as Naja.

Things I learnt from Scott

My kitchen became my canvas.

Chapter 20: When love came to my home

Hi Scott,

It was last Sunday, 27 February 2022. I was shopping at Woolworths, the local supermarket. I was feeling in a good mood.

At the till I had an impulse to buy a chocolate for the till lady. Truth be told I felt like a chocolate but that was a way to deal with it. She refused me so without being upset I turned around to the person behind me. I offered him a chocolate and he also refused it. Then he quickly said yes, as long as I would share it with him.

I waited on the bench at Woolies for him to finish his shopping. It was like a chocolate 'date' and there were even flutterings in my stomach. I was about to meet a total stranger.

It was such a rare thing to do and he and I were both laughing at this experience. We got on famously immediately and he kept saying I had to meet his wife. That afternoon all his family came to visit.

It was so absolutely wonderful. We were on the same page on many things. Including that we had all been at Canberra at the freedom rally at the same time. Not only had we arrived within the hour of each other we were camped in the same lane way, a few caravans apart.

Canberra's freedom rally was for me such a great experience of being surrounded by thousands of people experiencing a cause and a cry for freedom and love. A cry to stop the lunacy related to mandates and the nonsense of Covid laws.

Danni and Jimmy were a couple who depicted this love and freedom living it daily. I had invited into my house a family living in freedom and in love.

They had met when Jimmy advertised his house for rent. Danni arrived. He knew then she was for him. I don't think she did at that point. It took two weeks until the love blossomed and she became a non-paying renter.

Their opening statements to each other were to be kind to each other. And that, I say, is evident in their love of each other and the love through the family.

They left their stable life, including losing many close friends through the vaccination scam. They bought a caravan and let themselves be taken where-ever.

Jimmy's statement about me was, we are now friends for life; I feel it too. I feel honoured to know such a shining couple and to watch their journey unfold.

I cannot personally stop the bombs of the world but I can spread little bits of love through the Chocolate Love Revolution.

May more people buy a stranger a chocolate and spread the love.

It was, I guess, the beginning of me opening my house/self to allow love in.

I now have three new house mates. That is a very big step for me. Meeting the love of this experience.

This life I am living in the last few days feels as though I have stepped into a movie. A Fellini movie, divine weirdness.

The house is now a hub of laughter, spiritual bliss and joy. Netflix and the couch have retired and it is now interactions, cooking and eating with company.

Last night's meal was Mary's first one as a tenant in the house. I had made a big vegetable soup, seasoned with ginger, garam masala and cumin. I have found experimenting with seasonings in a small bowl works rather well. Of course, in this time my baking has flourished. In the last few days there have been carrot cakes, chocolate chip biscuits and chocolate treats.

Last night's dinner again was a magical experience. We have been having gatherings and parties most nights since the tenants moved in.

A young man Tim arrived with the tenants. He is somewhat an unusual young man of 21 years age. He gives the most loving hugs and is like an enthusiastic puppy dog.

By the way we all admit we are a strange bunch but we seriously are celebrating it. Literally from all different universes, dimension, planets and realities.

Tim is studying sound engineering at SAE.

The two male tenants were in the kitchen (my dream view), and Mary and I were enjoying watching them prepare the rest of the meal.

I suggested that Tim and I play a duet on the piano.

I don't know if words can express what happened. From the audience's perspective it sounded like we had been playing together for years.

From my perspective it was like the finest love making of my life. (And we know I have had a good few experiences...)

I literally was peaking and then quietening then peaking into another flow. When we started Tim had encouraged me to remember the pause - he related it to writing, that the full stops and commas were important. (In my early writing career they were really a nuisance and my editor did have a big task on her hands. I do believe I have now, 6 books later, improved.)

Of course, related to life, not just full steam ahead. In this new flow that is important as so much magic happens in one day.

Our movements, our flow, our connection via the keyboard was pure and utter bliss. Despite the fact that some of the keys on the piano were sticky and silent.

When we finished I said that was like making love. He agreed. I also asked him if that experience we had had is common and from what I gathered, it was a rare meeting.

Many laughs were had about the newly acquired flush I now had. All this interaction was taking place with my eyes closed and trusting my fingers on the keyboard. Is this the new metaphor for my life?

What was interesting is that Tim had stopped playing the piano for a year before. Just like I have stopped painting. It will be amazing to see what paintings I create when I start again. It is like fine wine -sometimes a resting period is needed.

Tim at 21 years old could be the most amazing lover, knowing that flow on the piano and translating it to a body must be amazing.

Guess I will never know as that, even for me, is too young.

I honour now that I am making love, however, in different ways. It has been pure magic the last few days. Talk about love coming in many forms.

I am loving living this love now. In forms that are not conventional, in dynamic flow, in this house that is buzzing with love, laughter and food.

Each day is a magical experience.

Love can come in many forms.

Things I learnt from Scott

Love wins.

Acknowledgement

To my editor and friend Jenni Gerrard, without you my writing would wilt.

To Scott Foster you helped lift a great weight off my shoulders. I am so grateful to you, you never waivered in your loving presence even when things were so tough.

To David B for helping me with the title and also being present for me when the crap hit the fan.

To the friends who had to wait for me, I am back.

ABOUT the author

Leeorah Hursky was born in South Africa .She has worked internationally as a healer and is also an artist. She resides in Australia now.

Books by Leeorah

I used to paint monsters

Naked Soul

Puppets on strings

Emotional Fat

How I lost my Mojo